SOME R

I found Karen's testimony of her healing journey ~~both inspiration~~ /ing. The authenticity and transparency in her heartfelt sharing will bring encouragement and hope to so many. It's the journey of moving from weakness to a powerful rediscovery of the depth of Father God's love. The security of that special place of rest and identity as a daughter in the Father's family brings.

We all can identify with those life experiences of wilderness and desperation. I believe Karen's story of her process, promptings, special prayers, and community will be a source of wisdom, encouragement, and hope to all in those desperate times when the supernatural power of a loving God is needed to bring restoration and rest in the midst of trial and challenge.

– Pastor Ken Hooper
Peninsula City Church, Frankston, Australia

These are extremely important books. They deal with one of the big questions in life: how do I deal with my pain? Whether it's physical or emotional pain, Karen's books will be the voice of a treasured friend who helps you through. Karen has shared her difficult journey of healing in a way that is easy to read, practical, full of encouragement and hope.

I pray they bless you as they have me; they are anointed, powerful and a treasure trove of wisdom.

– Deborah Lewis

Having known Karen for eighteen years and journeying closely with her over the past four years, I can attest to Karen's character and life. Karen lives what she speaks. This book and the wisdom it contains is gold for everyone, especially those with chronic illness. Do yourself a favor. Grab a copy and devour the insights Karen shares, and you'll receive hope and be transformed in the process.

– Jane Berry, Author
Ministering like Jesus: How to Grow
in Healing, Deliverance, and Miracles"
unlockingthegold.com

OMG! I absolutely love this! Cried my eyes out!

I can't wait to read the rest of the book…I now understand why it has taken so long to write. This is not something that could be rushed.

Love, Love, Love it! Good job!"

— Lisa Elliott

I found Karen's stories so uplifting and inspiring as I was experiencing a dry season in my life at the time of reading.

I've known Karen since she was a teenager, and she is such a gentle, kind soul who radiates Jesus' love. Her story is raw and honest. Her relationship with God is so beautiful.

Thank you Karen, for sharing your journey with us.

— Lynne Burgess, Author
All-In Night
All-In 2Night: Christian Activities for Families

"Be Still." This is difficult to do when you live in chronic pain. Karen challenges us to see God and trust Him in our waiting rooms. Her book and life will draw you to "Turn your eyes on Jesus."

— Debbie Patrick, Author
Founder of *Anchored and Alive*

Karen intuitively invites the reader to come alongside her as she vividly describes special encounters with God. Her sensitive writing allows us to sense God's presence and get lost in the moment. More than a memoir or devotional, this series of books showcase how intimately God notices us, begging us to be present, gently guiding us to notice Him—even during physical, mental, and emotional challenges.

Authentically, we learn to reach beyond our issues and love others, as we rely on the strength of the One who knows us inside and out.

— Susan Hoekstra, Author, Musician, Lay counsellor
A Firm GRASP: Feeling Validated in a Notice-Me World
Host of THE NOTICE podcast

BE *Held* BY *Him*

BOOK 1

BE *Held* BY *Him*

FINDING GOD WHEN LIFE KNOCKS YOU OFF YOUR FEET

KAREN BROUGH

Written by a very natural girl and a supernatural God

WRITTEN BY
God's girl

*Dedicated to those walking through
tough seasons right now.*

*You are not alone in all that you are experiencing.
He is closer to you than your breath, and
He cares more than you realize.*

You will get through this.

*And to my God and family, who carried
me when I couldn't do a thing.*

*I am so thankful for you and love you
more than you will ever know.*

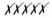

EDITOR

(The ultimate language artist, accomplished, generous, and precious new friend from across the oceans)

Linda Stubblefield | affordablechristianediting.com

GRAPHIC CONCEPT DESIGN

(The intuitive, talented creative heart and developer of dreams)

Abigail Parker | abigail@sponge.com.au

MAP ILLUSTRATOR

(The courageous, gifted, illustrative visionary and Holy Spirit led, heart woman of His)

Stacey Leitch | staceyleitch.com

BOOK COVER DESIGN & FORMATTING

(The oh so patient, professional, full of integrity, skilled book creative and design king)

Steve Kuhn | kuhndesigngroup.com

Contents

Foreword 11

Preface 17

Map 22

Introduction: *Where It All Began* 25

1. Rest: *What to Do When You Can't Do Anything* 35

2. Be Still: *One Solution to a Racing Mind* 47

3. Giving and Receiving: *But Needy Is Hard, Lord* 63

4. Atmosphere: *Your Environment Can Change You* 77

5. Never Alone: *Isolation Is a Lie* 93

6. Safe Places and Safe People: *Worthy of Safety* 109

7. Trust: *Dare to Trust Again* 125

8. Kindness: *Be Kind to Yourself* 139

9. God's Character: *God's Nature and Heart* 155

10. Listening: *Opening the Ears of My Heart* 169

11. God's Presence: *Life Is More than What Is Seen* 183

12. Prayer: *Developing Awareness of God in the Everyday* 195

13. Weakness: *When I Am Weak, He Is Strong* 211

14. Small Things: *Valuing the Small Builds the BIG* 227

15. Practical Survival Tips: *Life Checks and Balances* 241

16. Village Life: *Community—A Little Piece of Heaven* 257

For Those on a Spiritual Journey Who Want to
Connect with God for Themselves 271

Acknowledgments and Thankfest 277

About the Author 288

Foreword

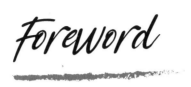

E ver since Karen mentioned to me she was writing a book; I've been excited to get my hands on it. Karen has immense authority when it comes to writing about the content this book addresses. She is a true overcomer in the face of adversity and ongoing crisis. Even if you do not share Karen's faith, there is something beautiful to read here.

Anyone who knows Karen would attest she is a very genuine, open, and authentic woman. Having demonstrated consistently over time an ability to live from a place of peace, despite her extraordinary and prolonged health crisis, means Karen is a voice worth listening to.

You see, I have known Karen for over fifteen years. I first met Karen when she was referred to see me from another local chiropractic practice. Karen's clinical presentation and health history were complex. Simply put, her body was a mess. She was in a health crisis. Even though I have assessed thousands of patients over the last 20 years, Karen's initial examination results are amongst those I still vividly recall. They don't stand out because they're good.

As a practitioner, I have seen my fair share of people in crisis. What fascinated me from my earliest years in practice, was trying to understand why some people are able to rise above their crisis while others are overwhelmed by it. I had observed that people with a faith background tended to fare better. But not always.

Even after only a handful of consultations, I remember being impressed with how sincere Karen was about her faith. I was encouraged that such a belief system may help her navigate the future that may lay ahead. However, I had some concerns. There was no doubt that to Karen, the existence of a miracle-breathing God was real. Unfortunately, given the reality of her medical condition, it seemed to me that Karen's medical condition and belief system were on a collision course.

I was afraid I was about to witness a train wreck. I had sadly seen this sort of thing play out before.

My concern for Karen was simple. Her condition and situation were not likely to improve; if that proved to be the case, would it eventually trigger a crisis of faith? How would she respond once she realized her 'miracle breathing God' was not providing her a miracle? Would Karen lose hope in her God? If so, would the trauma of a faith crisis further accelerate her downward health spiral?

In any case, it appeared to me that based on her health information alone, there would be tough days ahead.

What was perhaps unknown to Karen and her health care team was how much further her health would deteriorate. Indeed, her crisis deepened significantly. Insidiously, Karen completely lost her ability to work. Both her career and volunteering came to a grinding halt. Karen lost her ability to be active, socialize or even get out of the house. She would go on to experience multiple whole body collapses. It was evident to all that chronic disease was painfully and progressively stealing the best years of life away from this beautiful, intelligent, and caring woman.

This high-achieving woman and dedicated mother could no longer function. Period. Her former life stopped. Completely.

From a practitioner's perspective, Karen's story was in the top 1% of all clinical nightmares. It was a never-ending cycle of debilitating illness punctuated by excruciatingly painful flare-ups and a merry-go-round of doctor's appointments. As with many people with chronic health conditions, Karen suffered for a long time before getting a proper diagnosis. Sadly, once the diagnosis was established, Karen was confronted with the reality that while her condition was diagnosable, it was not medically curable. There was no 'wonder pill.' No magic bullet. No special diet. Nothing.

It is precisely this point that makes Karen's book so powerful and relevant.

Karen's journey is one of victory, like few people ever experience. It is not just about a deeply personal struggle with serious health issues. It is the lived experience of one who has overcome a crisis, even when the crisis is still ongoing. It is a story of finding peace, fulfillment, joy, and hope, even when your circumstances scream that it is impossible to do so. Even when you believe in miracles and no miracle of healing arrives in the expected or hoped for way.

What could be more relevant today than the real and personal experience of another human being who has faced a crisis and overcome.

Karen's book is not an account of her sickness. It is not a depressing read about one person's battle with failing health. It is not about her suffering. There is no chronological story telling from front to back cover. It is much more than that. Rather, it is almost as if Karen has generously opened up to us the most private pages in her journal and drawn out the nuggets of universal truth that have strengthened and encouraged her. Truths that have transformed her during, and even despite, her crisis.

It is a deep dive of discovery into the essence of what it means to be a human being. Karen has been vulnerable and brave. Raw and real. She has not held back. She has done more than just share her personal insights and reflections. She has provided us a road map based on her lived experience. A road map we can apply on our own journey of discovery to finding peace, fulfillment, joy, and hope. Even when life hurts.

This book is a wonderful resource. I would encourage you to read it the way it has been intended. Sit and ponder a chapter at a time. Even just part of a chapter. The book has been designed to choose the order in which you read the chapters, feel free to skip about in the book, allow yourself to be encouraged, uplifted, challenged, and stirred.

Unlike Karen, your crisis may not be a health crisis. Yours might be financial. Or relational. Or mental. Maybe your life has been interrupted by tragedy or an unexpected accident. Perhaps a loved one has been torn from you. You may have suffered abuse, isolation, or judgment. Whatever the case, this book is relevant to you. Karen has skillfully lifted the gems of truth from her own experience and has presented them to us here in a kindly and caring manner. What she shares is relevant to us no matter what crisis we face.

Perhaps your personal crisis hasn't even hit yet. Then all the better. You are in a wonderful and privileged position to dive into this book. Why wait for a crisis to discover greater meaning and richness in life.

One thing is sure, if you live long enough, you will experience your own personal crisis. Hopefully, yours is limited to a season in your life. Hopefully, yours ends in a miracle. But, whatever the case will be for you when your crisis comes, be encouraged that there will be a way forward.

This book makes a wonderful contribution to the understanding of how to transition from living as a "human doing" to becoming a completely fulfilled "human being." Karen authentically demonstrates that when you discover the richness of what it means to be a human being, being one is wonderful, despite your circumstance.

Karen's authentic life has touched me, my staff, and other patients. Despite her own serious medical battles, she has found the energy to write many kind, encouraging, inspired, and insightful personal notes to us over the years. I am now thrilled she has offered up this book into the public domain, where she shares with us openly the source of her strength. May this book enrich you in the way that Karen enriches those that know her.

Dr. Norman Craig Nelson
Chiropractor
BAppSc(ClinSc)/BChiropracticSc

Preface

Are you stressed, sick, worn out, or weary? Has your body broken, slowed up, or let you down?

Has life tossed you into unfamiliar waters, and you are struggling to find a place to land?

Do you feel out of control—at the whim of whatever comes at you, longing for something secure and unchanging to grab a hold of?

To feel "normal" again?

Have you ever felt that the situation you are facing is bigger than what you have the capacity to meet?

Do you feel as if you've nothing left to give, no ability to "push through" anymore?

Do you ever wonder where your peace and hope have gone, asking whether they're in hiding or have disappeared altogether?

Do you feel alone in all that you are walking through?

DO YOU FEEL ALONE IN ALL THAT YOU ARE WALKING THROUGH?

Have you ever thought, "Where are You, God? Why is this happening to me?"

Are you struggling to hear, see or connect with God?

Have you ever wanted to experience Him tangibly? To see and feel His miraculous touch, to hear His loving voice, to sit with Him in the barbed times of life, and have your wounds tended by Him?

If you've asked any or all of these questions, you're in good company, and this book is for you.

This is the book I needed ten years ago when I was struck with a debilitating mystery illness. Floundering for the first few months, I eventually realized that I needed God's help; the only way forward was with Him.

My offering is not intended to be a definitive final work on how and who God is; rather, a journey of one woman's encounter with Him in the hard places of tough seasons. Sharing the encouragements He poured out to me in these times, hoping they will speak to and reassure others as they experience their own hard times.

In seasons of life, increasing numbers of people find themselves facing fatigue and health breakdown. Stressors and trouble pile one upon another with minimal recovery time. Have you noticed it too? Have you felt it yourself?

The pace of life events, traumas, sicknesses have sought to push us away

- From our peace

- From one another

- From intimacy with God

- From the very things that would help us in these times.

The need to connect with the One who knows the way forward is essential to survive and thrive through whatever life throws at us—choosing to look through His lens rather than my limited vision.

Learning how to hear and see His heart for my circumstance brings a whole other level of hope. I don't know about you, but I need His vision so much, especially when life throws me into deep waters.

If we are to have hope and help in our hour of need, we need to know how to hear and recognize God's voice—not because we *should* do it but because we *get to*. His voice is worth listening to, and His heart brings us good at this time—every time.

As you read this book, you will be:

- Tended to by His loving words

- Reassured that you are not alone in your pain, grief, or trouble

- Encouraged that others have gone before you and survived

- Lighter, with seeds of hope planted deep within you

- Experiencing His helping, healing hand at work in the everyday moments of your life

- Observing the ordinary becoming extraordinary as you become more aware of Him

- Aware of His redemptive plans and purposes, reigniting hope within you

- Uplifted as you develop a greater connection to Father God and recognize the loving tones of His voice

I needed these helps when all seemed confusing, hopeless, and overwhelming. So much mystery surrounded the present and the future, and I felt despair as a result. As time wore on, I understood that I was unwilling to live without hope, and the only place I found lasting hope was with Him. The only way forward was to allow God to carry me through these initial stages of life's upheaval.

> I WAS UNWILLING TO LIVE WITHOUT HOPE, AND THE ONLY PLACE I FOUND LASTING HOPE WAS WITH HIM

Go on a journey together with Him. He won't load you down with more burdens but instead, lighten the load you already carry, healing and tending to raw spaces along the way.

Come. Come and be encouraged by God and all that He has done. Be uplifted, knowing that what He does for one, He can do for you and more.

LETTER TO THE READER

Dear Precious One Walking through a Time of Rough and Tough,

I felt led to pen you a personal note of encouragement. I pray that this little book will bring you some hope. That your current circumstance won't define you but be a springboard for something better—even while army crawling through it!

Here are just a handful of the stories, experiences, and encouragements that God poured out upon me during my own challenging time. He has made this past decade-long chronic health challenge all the sweeter for having met Him in the depths.

Even when my garden was engulfed with weeds and filled with fertilizer stench, He has helped me see and smell the roses within it.

He is ready to help you to find a sweet aroma also.

I pray that you will be compelled to discover the *More* of God in this time—the depths of His heart of love for you personally. That you'll be forever changed for the better as a result of this season.

I pray that not a single day will go by where you don't encounter the sweetness of His embrace, the thrill of an adventure with Him, and reminders of how precious you are to Him.

I pray for God to strengthen and uplift you today. That today, you would know, is not too hard for you because He is with you always.

With much love and prayers for you during this time,

Karen
XXXXX

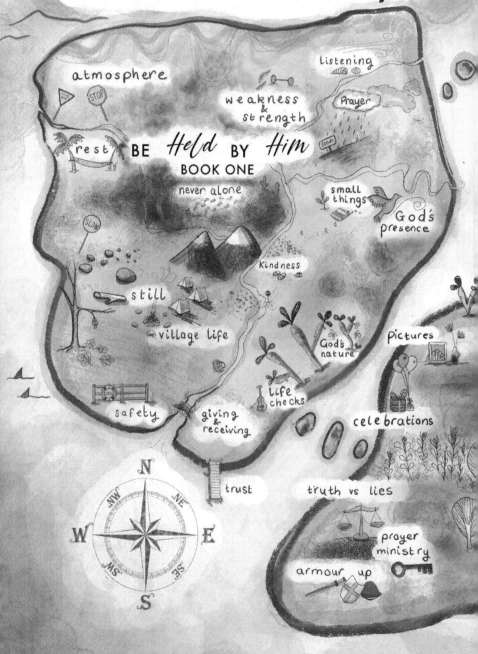

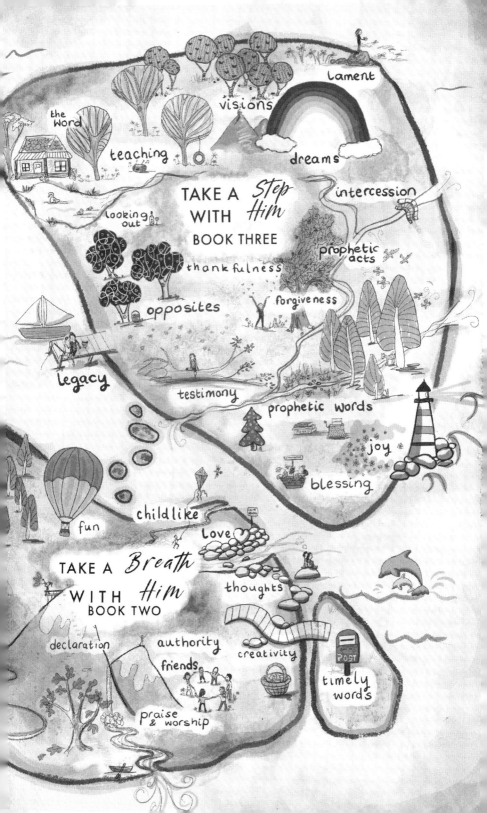

EXPLANATION OF THE MAP

'The Journey' map outlines the various chapters of each book in the 'Be Held by Him' series.

Rather than list off the chapter topics, the precious Mindy Kirker 'Flourish writers' suggested an infographic map might be effective in covering the content of the three books in one. It felt as if air came into my lungs when she suggested this God inspired idea. Thank-you Mindy!

Not long after this, God gave me a dream, revealing the three stages of health/capacity, when hardship hits. He revealed there were three islands, and just as I did, my reader would move from a desert like experience to places of flourish with Him.

Finally, through another dream, and a few recommendations from people in the dream, He brought across my path the gifted illustrator, Stacey Leitch. She understood the subject matter personally and the moment we spoke, I knew she would be the right person for the work.

She has created this prophetic artwork based on the book chapters and content. We've brainstormed and she's brought the conversations, God's instruction and her vision into something that continues to speak to me daily. God bless you and your gift Stacey.

'The Journey' reveals a story of how God speaks to and interacts with us, especially in the hard seasons of life. I've thoroughly enjoyed the detailed gifts of hope Stacey has helped communicate through the map and more than that, revealed Father's heart for us in the tough.

I pray it encourages you & invests hope in you.

There is always so much more to look forward to, with God by your side. Don't give up!

Introduction

"I am the branches; you are the leaf.

Come, connect to My life-giving branches once again.

Let Me pour life back into you.

Let Me restore your color.

Let Me hold you once again.

*My arms are open wide and ready to
embrace your battle-weary form.*

*In the natural, a young leaf is green, full of hope and
life. The elements seem to come relentlessly. Eventually,
the wind, rain, and storms wear it down, and the
now colorless, frail leaf falls from the tree lifeless.*

But with Me, this isn't the end, but the beginning.

I am counter-cultural and counter-intuitive.

*Where you may feel that your situation
has sucked the best years from you.*

That all is hopeless.

That there is no coming back from this place of upheaval.

Take heart, with Me, this is not the case.

*You come to Me, dry, brittle, worn out and weary,
and I begin to pour Myself into those desert places.*

As you are held by Me, I pour My life into you.

I apply balm to your trodden, wilderness areas.

I restore your color.

I give you back life and bright eyes.

I lead you to green places of flourish.

*Where the world saps the life from you,
I give you life and life to the full.*

*Take heart, My precious one; I am not limited by what you
see or feel—there is HOPE and much future to be had.*

You can come back from this and thrive with Me.

*My beloved, this isn't the end of you, but the
beginning of something new in you as you
allow Me to embrace you once again."*

———————

"How does an autumn leaf relate to being held?

I think you just answered me, Father. Thank You."

EACH CHAPTER CONTAINS
THE FOLLOWING ELEMENTS:

1. **A Key for hardship** (chapter title)

   God gave me each one, showing me their importance in faith and surviving hard seasons.

2. **Testimony**

   God highlighted how He had been in the middle of so many experiences in the depths. These stories testify to His goodness.

3. **Father's heart about each key**

   God's encouragement taken from my journals as He responded to my questions and shared with me about the keys.

4. **Prayer**

A quick proviso:

You might notice as you read that I don't use the traditional term "the Holy Spirit." This is a personal thing for me, and by no means do I wish to cause offense to anyone who thinks differently.

Each part of God—Father, Jesus, and Holy Spirit- is tangible, alive, and personable. Each is complete in themselves, but each connects with me in different ways.

For me to address "Holy Spirit" as "the Holy Spirit" would be to hold Him at a distance, and I want Him as near as possible. Please feel free to add "the" if that designation fits with how you communicate with Him.

Bless you, precious one. *XXXXX*

A Word of Warning

The following is my personal "beginning" health story that could contain some triggering aspects for those in raw places.

If you are in this place, you may want to consult the contents page for a chapter that speaks directly to your heart.

WHERE IT ALL BEGAN

Lying upon the bed, unable to move my limbs, head, and body, my heart wept. *Am I dying? Is this IT? What about my hubby Craig and the kids?* Thoughts were racing in and out, endeavoring to find a place to land, to find order and explanation…but at that moment, there was none to find.

The constant headache of the past six weeks hadn't slowed me up; I pushed through, taking paracetamol to try and ease the knifelike pangs, to no avail. I pushed on, meeting the commitments, the pressures of being a wife, a mum, a business partner, a teacher, the various voluntary committees, responsibilities, and relationships—everything cried out for more—of me. That small voice within screamed for me to slow down, but in my mind, there was simply no time…

MY BODY HAD HAD ENOUGH! I NOW HAD NO CHOICE; MY BODY WOULD TAKE WHAT IT NEEDED – WITH OR WITHOUT MY PERMISSION.

No time to stop…

No time to consider and ask what was causing the unfamiliar symptom…

No time to cull the calendar craziness…

No time to be still…

No time…

No time…

No time…

"It'll have to wait" was a common thought of this time, prioritizing everyone else but myself. Sacrificing myself for others, that's what real service is about, isn't it? I was a servant-hearted wife of one, the mother of three, and now I couldn't do a thing.

My body had sent out the warning signs—the unheeded flashing red lights trying their best to let me know things weren't right. I hadn't listened, and now, I'd pushed it beyond its limits. Layer upon layer of the past year's stresses flooded to mind as I lay there, waiting for the ambulance to arrive.

Pale, exhausted, unable to lift a single finger, I was at the whim of life and circumstances. My body had had enough! I now had no choice; my body would take what it needed—with or without my permission.

So, I lay there, so filled with weakness that nothing would function as I willed it to—as fear expanded within.

Terror seized my distress, and they embraced.

As the seconds passed, new symptoms appeared, and I felt as though life was leaving me. My eyes closed, and I tried desperately to come to peace with what I was leaving behind.

My family, oh, my precious family—Craig, my children.

Just moments before, in our first extended family dinner in months, we had been busy catching up around the dinner table. Everyone was able to be there; what a delight! So good to be back at the family home.

Squeals of joy came from our kids and their cousins as they played happily in the background. Mum and Dad were in the kitchen cleaning up, and my sister and I bantered back and forth across the table, having some good hearty laughs. These times were precious. My family was so dear to me. Together is the place I wanted to be all the time. These nights were a balm for my soul.

Then in a split second, everything changed.

My eyes began to move of their own accord as if some mysterious fingers were pulling the muscles behind them. My neck became sore, stiff, and the slight headache intensified.

My body felt the waves of nausea and fatigue HIT, and boy, did it hit! Any energy I had dissipated and withdrew, heading who knows where. Beginning with my extremities, I felt as if my blood was retreating. My hands weakened, and my arms fell limply to the sides of my body. My head joined the procession and dropped upon my shoulder. The weightiness of it propelled my immobilized body to the right—where Craig sat.

"Catch me, honey," I barely breathed out as my entire body fell upon his lap.

Apart from the sheer physical exhaustion and my brain feeling as though it was splitting in two, I don't remember much of the following minutes. My listless, unresponsive form was carried to my parent's bedroom nearby, and an ambulance was called.

Time stood still, and I couldn't comprehend much of what anyone was saying. Every cell of my body felt weighty—sleepy, as if the energy had been sucked out of every molecule. They demanded rest, and rest they did.

The medical staff arrived, and the family tension was relieved on some level for a moment. The cavalry had arrived, and now they could "fix" Karen.

They took my vitals and eventually surmised that I was "…just a tired Mum" as they offered to take me into the hospital but articulating that they wouldn't do much for me in the hospital. Confusion…upset…shock remained.

Ever so slightly, a minuscule amount of strength found its way to my extremities, and my limbs began to be able to move once again. They felt weighty and slow-moving—like I was on heavy medication or in recovery from surgery. But the exhaustion remained.

A NEW SEED OF AFFLICTION AND FEAR HAD BEEN PLANTED THAT NIGHT AND WOULD ENDEAVOR TO WREAK HAVOC IN OUR LIVES FOR MANY MONTHS AND YEARS TO COME.

I remember Craig asking what I wanted to do. I remember not wanting to or being able to decide. My brain had ceased to be able to think coherently. The decision was made not to go to the hospital, and as the ambulance officers left, the hope of help seemed to depart with them.

Inside, my questions mounted, *How could they leave me here like this? What was going to happen?*

Soon after, we headed home as if nothing had happened.

The only thing was something HAD happened and was indeed happening.

My body had never felt such fatigue before. It was as if I'd been hit by a Mack truck or run a 100km marathon in a moment. Every part of me ached and screamed, "I'm so weary."

I remained silent. No one spoke on the way home. The fear was palpable, and no one knew what to say. Ours was the quietest car trip our family had ever had.

The sounds of the tires on the road hurt my head; the glare of the streetlights stung my eyes. Sitting upright was a challenge as my head felt like a bowling ball. As we rattled along, my head leaned against the cold passenger window. Every bump, every knock, every turn felt and intensified. This was the longest car trip I'd ever had.

I plopped into bed, desperate for sleep. My eyelids closed as a signal for sleep to come, but it evaded me much of that night.

Fearful thoughts raced around and persisted for hours as the shock and trauma of what had occurred replayed inside my head. A new seed of affliction and fear had been planted that night and would endeavor to wreak havoc in our lives for many months and years to come.

The next morning, I woke, meaning I must've slept, but I felt no benefit, no refreshment or energy. My eyelids were heavy; my brain matter felt as if it was crystallizing inside like crackling ice as the temperature warms. So too was my head and its sensitivity to every-thing. The whole-body weakness persisted, and I struggled to stand, to talk, or to walk upright.

A barrage of thoughts tried to rattle my weary frame. *You have a brain tumor. You're going to die a slow, painful death. Your family will see it and be powerless. It'll be painful for them too. It's going to get worse*, and many more.

I was in the space of sheer terror; my pupils dilated almost wholly, and my snowlike complexion showed that things were not as they should be. Something was desperately wrong, and I was without solutions.

I felt a small and insignificant voice in a body that refused to obey my commands anymore.

I don't remember thinking of or speaking to God much during this time; I allowed fear to reign mostly in this space.

All I could squeak out in a moment of reprieve was a single word…"Help!"

He heard my cry, and help came.

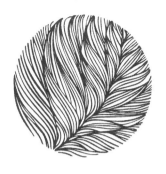

Chapter One

REST

And He said, "My Presence will go with you, and I will give you rest."

EXODUS 33:14 NKJV

There I sat, contemplating all that had happened over the past couple of years.

How did I get to this place where life as I once knew it was unrecognizable...endeavoring to make sense of all that had happened and trying desperately to formulate a plan that would restore my capacity to be all that I had once been.

On this day, I sat on the daybed, looking out to the garden and road in front of me. I noticed the bounty of flowers, the bees going about their business of taking pollen from one flower to the next. They had a life. They knew their job. They could do all they were created to do. Their life was simple, straightforward.

How I envied them.

The local road signs were highlighted to me as my eyes wandered across the scape. If my life had signposts, they would read ANXIETY, PAIN, CONFUSION, FEAR.

I sat pondering all the medical mysteries and mountains of worry. In my weakness, my mind regularly raced without reprieve, focusing upon all I had lost…grieving my career…my sense of identity…my strength…my former life and ability to do something—anything.

"Where are You, Lord?" my heart cried from the depths. Painfully aware of how my lack was weighing upon the lives of others, my symptoms remained. My inner world trembled in turmoil, living with three tensions:

- Frustration at not being who I once was

- Learning to be at peace when there was so much mystery.

- If I wasn't me anymore, who was I now?

"Rest, My child."

He lovingly waited on me.

I had been so strong for so long. A "normal" busy Mum in Australian society, engaging with the relentless flow of demands and "good" things. Regularly pushing myself for others who were in need.

"This was how we were meant to live, wasn't it, Lord? Don't You want me to do good things? Why is this happening to me?" The questions came thick and fast, and mostly without answers.

Without enough energy to process solutions, I really wasn't interested in hearing any answers…

I poured out of my "lack" well and found it was a deep, cavernous space.

He patiently listened. He wasn't shaken by my questioning.

I sat weeping as I journaled, pouring it all out to Him—day after day, week after week.

He gently spoke refreshing words of hope to me.

God began showing His personal life signs for me. They were distinctly different than those I had chosen for myself. They read:

"Stop."

"Wait."

"Be Still."

"Rest in Me."

I didn't understand these words. Life was busy. Everyone around me was busy.

Like most in our circle of friends, we had been "living the dream." Hindsight is a beautiful intangible. As I brought these observations to Father, new seeds of truth were planted. The truth being, we were overloaded with good things but rarely able to take a moment to enjoy any of them.

Busy with everyone, connecting with few. Being the answer rather than pointing to the One who is the answer.

Busy with everyone, connecting with few.

My heart had always desired more, but there simply wasn't time to ask why I continued doing the good when God's best was available to me.

WE WERE OVERLOADED WITH GOOD THINGS BUT RARELY ABLE TO TAKE A MOMENT TO ENJOY ANY OF THEM.

So the calendar remained full. Serving others on fumes continued until I couldn't "do" anything anymore.

All busyness gave me was more of the same. Unquenchable flames roaring out of control, licking up every bit of fuel they can absorb. Never satisfied—never enough until all capacity is gone. Leaving a desolate wasteland in its wake.

REST

Is this it, Lord? Is this all that life is meant to be—a constant state of expectations and boxes? Surely there's more?

The model around me was life success meant independence, personal ability, physical strength, do, do, do.

No time to be.

No time to pick up rest.

Could it be that You see this differently, Lord?

> **ALL BUSYNESS GAVE ME WAS MORE OF THE SAME.**

Could it be that You have something different in mind for me? Something that doesn't look like other's journeys?

He brought to mind the snapshots of life events of the past—indicators that the path I was on wasn't the right one for me or my design.

Two weeks before moving house, schools, and life, we held a thankyou lunch for over one hundred family and friends. People arrived, ate, and conversed as their kids played. I barely remember anything about it.

Floating through the lunch. I don't recall a single conversation. As lunch became dinner for a few, I sat zombie-like inside. Crashing into bed at the end of the day. Requiring days of recovery, but not having them available. Indicative of my inner state. Buzzing through life, ticking off the "to-do" lists. No wiggle room, no margins—nothing but a fast-paced well of ever asking.

As I pondered this memory, I noted my joy had gone into hiding, and I consistently felt on edge. *Why hadn't I noticed?*

As I sat on the daybed, now months after the lunch…the days seemed to turn into weeks. It had been such an intense season.

"It won't be too much longer, Karen; hang in there," I told myself.

But the reality is, I'd been saying that for about twelve months, and there was still no end in sight.

It was the collapse. Only when my body physically fell to pieces, was I able to stop. There was no other option. Nothing was left in the tank for my body to draw upon.

In a single moment, there was no more pushing through—no more busyness…no more racing here and there—only the feeling of nothing.

After such a busy time of fast-paced seasons, I now had an abundance of what I craved throughout it all—time.

Time to think…

Time to worry…

Time to ponder…

Time to question…

As friends and family continued to bring me gifts from God of time, care, and all that was needed, this season became one of learning how to receive. I'd been a giver all my life, but God wanted to give me gifts. And to learn how to rest, I needed help. I needed others. I needed Him. It was my time to receive the gift of resting in Him.

Page after page, I filled journals with questions, griefs, and processings with God. Some days writing pages, others, a single word.

> HE LOVINGLY RESPONDED WITH ALL I NEEDED TO HEAR AT THAT MOMENT.

He lovingly responded with all I needed to hear at that moment.

"Rest, My child."

REST

"Rest, My child."

"Who am I, if I can't do anything, Lord?"

He encouraged me, gently responding, *"My beloved, life is complete as you choose to walk hand in hand with Me. It was never designed to be about what you do for Me alone."*

As I rested before Him, I felt peaceful—more peaceful than I had felt in months.

Hope was watered.

If I was with God, then everything else shrank, and the heaviness lightened.

I longed to remain in rest because of what it brought to me in my time of need.

In the rest I was hearing God more.

In the rest He reassured me.

In the rest my fears were relieved.

Rest was the place where even though physically weak, I became strong with Him.

Then Jesus said, "Let's go off by ourselves to a quiet place and rest awhile." He said this because there were so many people coming and going that Jesus and his apostles didn't even have time to eat.

MARK 6:31 NLT

Come to me all who are weary and burdened, and I will give you rest. Take my yoke upon you and learn from me, for I am gentle and humble in heart, and you will find rest for your souls. For my yoke is easy, and my burden is light.

MATTHEW 11:28-30 NIV

— Father's Heart —

My rest is an inner peace that remains whatever may come.

My rest refreshes the inner man so that the outer man can walk fearlessly forward into the plans I have for them.

My rest is the meeting place between you and Me.

It is where My Spirit speaks, and you hear Me.

It is a perfect place of communion: you and I walking together as we were designed to.

My rest can be taken up or put down.

Walking in My rest is a choice.

I will never force My rest upon you, child, because My will is for you to choose Me—out of love.

In My rest, the cares and worries of the world do not burden you as heavily because I give you the resources of heaven and kingdom perspective.

In that place you and I accomplish unimaginable things while we simply be with one another.

Stop for a moment, child.

*I call you **child** because no matter how old you may feel, compared to Me, you are always young, full of life, full of purpose, and full of My hope.*

Pick up My peace and regain My rest.

Now walk forward in it.

If you find yourself overwhelmed or in fear, stop once more and take up My rest once again.

Are you weary, tired, burnt out?

Do you struggle to stop and be still?

I am.

I am here.

I am here for you, and I have wonderful truths to pour upon you in your wilting state.

Take heart; you will stand tall once again.

What you walk now is not the end but the beginning of something even more beautiful than before.

Come; let's walk a while, and I will bring you rest.

REST

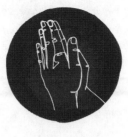

— *Prayer* —

Precious Father, my place of pure rest,

Thank You for Your permission to rest.

*Thank You that You promise when I am
weary or burdened, You will give me rest.*

*Thank You for everything You are to me and
all that You bring to me through rest.*

*I love that You long to show me how to abide
in rest, showing me how Your yoke is easy
and Your burden is light. It is refreshing!*

I feel hopeful as I rest.

*Thank You, Father, that You do not burden
me with more than I can carry.*

*You encourage me to pause, take life in, pick up
Your rest, and then go forward in true peace.*

Amen.

XXXXX

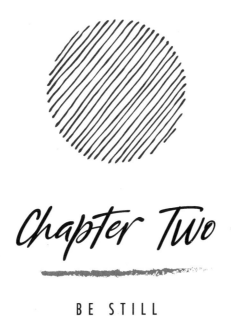

Chapter Two

BE STILL

The LORD will fight for you; you need only to be still.

EXODUS 14:14 NIV

Sitting in the vinyl chair, I wait for my name to be called. The room was busy; people were scurrying here and there—coming in and out. My body seemed to pick up on the intensity all around.

The phone's endlessly ringing. Reception staff speaking. In the corner, the morning television show blares mindless words that can't quite be heard over the hum in the room. Fluorescent lightbulbs are seeming to suck what little energy I have left from me.

Stop it, Lord, please stop it. It's too much. My heart cried out for some peace, some respite, some quiet.

"Be still, My child."

Only days earlier, He had said the same thing to me. In fact, it had been a frequent response to my heartfelt cries.

I'd been so unwell on that day. It had been a couch day when I had been unable to move or do much of anything. I remember feeling like my body had failed me. I hated my system at times.

I REMEMBER FEELING LIKE MY BODY HAD FAILED ME. I HATED MY SYSTEM AT TIMES.

It was supposed to be able to push through—to support my life-style—not govern it! I longed for it to be better. *How I wish you were a healthier and stronger body!* Spurts of tears and emotional out-bursts came forth.

I sat on our front deck, desperate for my body to be repaired by someone. It simply wasn't happening.

My brain strived to be able to think coherently once more, but I found thinking too painful. Constant fog-like flu and knifelike pains zapped my brain without warning.

Pain is exhausting.

So I endeavored to sleep, to rest.

"Be still, My child."

But I have so much I need to be doing.

"This is your time to be still. Let others take care of things for a while."

I don't like being still. It's awkward and difficult. It feels unnatural to my buzzing system. My brain races. My body races too.

Am I ever going to get better, Lord?

"It's in the 'Be still' that you will heal."

I don't feel like me. Who am I—if I can't do anything?

"You could sit on this couch for the rest of your life, and I could not love you any more or less."

*But…but…but…*the excuses and questioning continued.

At the same time, I endeavored to process all that He was saying.

So, I asked Him, "How could You love me if I sit and do nothing?"

*"I care far more about your **being** than your **doing**. It's in the **being** with Me that you can do. Be still, My child, and rest."*

Back in the waiting room, as I looked around, I saw the downcast, wrinkled, and weary faces. Affliction seemed all around me.

A mother tried unsuccessfully to soothe her crying baby. I couldn't even feign care; nothing—no capacity to help—seemed left inside of me—not even a small nod. I had no energy to give her an encouraging "I understand" or "You'll get there." This inability was so unlike me. I didn't recognize myself some days.

When is this all going to end? The anxiety built as the angst in the room sought to steal from me what little peace I had left.

"YOU COULD SIT ON THIS COUCH FOR THE REST OF YOUR LIFE, AND I COULD NOT LOVE YOU ANY MORE OR LESS."

"Breathe in, breathe out."

This was yet another pathology room experience—clinical. Cold. Compounding a feeling of impersonal processing of brokenness and weakness, I hated these places.

Get me out of here! Oh, Lord, I'm anxious; this whole scene scares me. Help!

"Close your eyes, My child."

I let my lids close ever so gently.

In a room that felt harsh and intense, I took a moment to stop, listen, and obey. It was a welcome relief.

What next?

"Rest....be still. Let all your body parts learn the rhythm of 'be still' with me."

BE STILL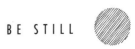

I found myself counting as I slowed my breathing.

My internal racing began to settle.

The thoughts and absorption of all that was around me seemed to fade away. As He stilled my heart and mind. It was as if the noise from outside, disappeared.

Oh, God, thank You.

Becoming more aware of His stillness and His presence in the quiet, His "be still" became more significant than anything else around me.

> TAKING A DEEP BREATH, I PICKED UP HIS "BE STILL." SENSING LIKE I WAS NOW TEFLON-COATED TO FEAR.

In that space, I found myself letting go of fear…letting go of the overwhelm—merely being in the moment.

No lights. No sound. No expectation of answers or questions—just merely being with God.

The quick-paced tone of my heart was now calm, stable, and predictable.

Oh, Lord, can I remain here? I love this. Thank You.

The outside world had melted away as I spent time with Him.

Time passed by…who knows how long. Seconds? Minutes? Hours? There was no rush here, and with all the physical symptoms I'd experienced on this average morning, this "be still" was a welcome new friend.

"Karen? Karen Brough?" The nurse called out from the blood-sucking room.

My eyes shot open, and I acknowledged her with a wave. I rose to my feet, feeling as though I'd had a refreshing sleep. Step by step, I could still feel the residue of that "be still" moment.

How wonderful this is, Lord!

As I approached the beige double doors with Pathology written in bold, black-printed letters, fear tried to sneak back in. I felt it knocking at the entrance of my mind. Taking a deep breath, I picked up His "be still." sensing like I was now Teflon-coated to fear.

This is amazing!

Sitting now in the chunky beige chair with the enormously wide arms, I rolled up my sleeve. I sat, feeling sturdy and ready for whatever was to come. The nurse and I began to talk.

"So, what have you been experiencing? How did this happen?" The questions came thick and fast. Surprisingly, the answers came quickly and without effort. The flow of conversation was laced with hope and life.

The specifics are now a mystery to me.

I found myself encouraging this woman who was going through some tough things of her own.

God knew.

But as I spoke what came to mind, her mouth stood motionless, open, as God gave life words that spoke directly to her heart. Her eyes welled up at what God had given me to share—just for her.

How is this happening, Lord? She told me how she felt I'd been sent to her. She told me she was feeling much better about her situation.

"You have been battling so much, and yet you are so positive. How do you do that?" she asked, wide-eyed and ready to hear the answer—as if to say, "I need some of that; what's your secret?"

For a split second, I remembered how I'd been just minutes before in the waiting room. I was completely unqualified to answer these

BE STILL

questions. Then swiftly remembered how God had brought me to that beautiful, peaceful place.

"It's a God thing. He gives me so much to live for—even when the tough comes," I found myself responding.

He was encouraging me as much as she. You could've knocked me over with a feather as I heard myself speaking. *Wasn't I broken? What could I possibly bring to anyone at this time?* And yet, here I was. God had again done something miraculous.

His "be still" posture had come with me into that room, allowing all else to melt away—if but for a moment—to enable me to be present with this precious woman. She didn't yet know how much she was loved by Him.

She felt His peace. She was moved by His heart.

And I watched on from the sidelines in awe of Him and what He was doing.

The needle went in, and the blood was drawn almost effortlessly because the conversation was precious and distracting. She continued about her paperwork, stopping for moments. She asked questions and revealed more about her heart and journey.

The more we spoke, the more touched by God she was, and the more blessed and energized I felt.

God, You amaze me. How I can be so afflicted and in pain...and yet You've brought me here so that You could encourage this woman and strengthen me in the process. How does it happen?

Such a precious moment in time. Thank You for letting me be here today.

"You've got such peace about you. It's been so lovely to talk with you, Karen. I won't forget this. Thank you so much." Her last words to me uplifted me as I headed out of the room with a big smile on my face, eyes feeling light and refreshed. Body upright and heart about to burst with delight at what God had just done.

HOW DOES HE TURN AN AWFUL BEGINNING INTO AN ENLIGHTENED ENDING?

The lights weren't so bright.

The sounds were quieter in the waiting room.

The baby was sleeping in the pram beside its Mother.

I smiled at the downtrodden faces who looked at me. And they lifted as I walked towards reception.

How does God do this?

How does He turn an awful beginning into an enlightened ending?

It all begins with His "be still."

> Be still and know that I am God; I will be exalted among the nations; I will be exalted in the earth.
>
> **PSALM 46:10 NIV**

BE STILL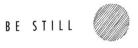

— Father's Heart —

Rush, rush, rush is what I see. Are you tired, beloved?
Are you weary? Do you find yourself desiring
rest but don't have a moment to yourself?

Come to Me. Come to Me, and I will
give you rest (Matthew 11:28).

Stop focusing on doing and just be—before Me. When
you are with others, it can often be like you are on
a treadmill—always moving, talking, doing, or
thinking about what you have to do—barely stopping.
Simply being present in the moment is rare.

When you are with Me, stop; be still.

Let your body rest before Me.

Let your mind rest for a bit.

Stop yourself from focusing on doing and just be—before
Me. Take some deep breaths and drink in My rest for you.
You might need to fight the tendency to talk or think or do.
With Me, you don't need to do anything at this moment.

Initially, it may not be easy to step into being still.

Often your day is so busy that your body and mind are working overtime. So many tasks to complete and people to care for. Let Me reassure you, My child, there will always be an endless list of tasks and people who have needs.

This moment right now will never be again. Let's enjoy a moment together in the practice of being still.

In My presence, you can be refreshed and renewed.

"Be still" is the place to pick up My peace. You can then go out and have a clear perspective, make wise decisions, and travel with Me through the day, feeling lighter.

When you come to be still with Me, you are allowing Me to talk to you. Within the still, it will not be overwhelming or busy, but a rewarding time of filling.

Be still and just listen to whatever My Spirit reveals.

*The **still** will sometimes be tangible thoughts and answers, but often it is merely about a Spirit-to-spirit time of just being. Soaking in more of who I am reveals a greater measure of Myself in you.*

My presence is full of peace for your battle-worn emotions.

My presence is love and acceptance when all around you cries out for more. My presence is joy when all around you seek to bring you down.

Doesn't being in My presence sound refreshing to you? Come; come to me, child, and be still before me. Offer Me a sacrifice of time, and I will make it the best investment of your day. Your life requires daily refreshment, and I am the answer to that need.

BE STILL

*Come now, tell Me of your worries, your dreams, and
your cares. Then stop, be still, rest, and listen.*

*Trust Me to bring all that you need for the
day ahead. Trust Me because I love you.*

*My beloved, it brings Me great joy when
you choose to come and be still.*

But they that wait upon the LORD shall renew their strength;
they shall mount up with wings as eagles; they shall run,
and not be weary; and they shall walk, and not faint.

ISAIAH 40:31 KJV

He got up, rebuked the wind and said
to the waves, "Quiet! Be still!"

Then the wind died down and it was completely calm.

He said to his disciples, "Why are you so
afraid? Do you still have no faith?"

They were terrified and asked each other, "Who is
this? Even the wind and the waves obey him!"

MARK 4:39-41 NIV

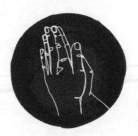

— *Prayer* —

Peace filling Jesus, Holy Spirit, and Father,

*The world around me has many distractions and
needs at times, being still can be challenging.*

*You have said that You want me to learn
the power of being still before You.*

Help me to learn this rhythm with You.

*Thank You for knowing what I need most and
bringing it to me during these times of stillness.*

I trust You when You say, You will strengthen me.

You will give me rest.

You will fight for me.

All I need to do is be still.

*I look forward to developing a rhythm of being still
that remains, connecting us in sweet abide.*

Only in You do I find my foundation for joy.

In the "be still" I feel more complete and at ease.

There You speak life over me, and I am postured to accept it.

Please take my hand and lead me into
that still, peaceful place with You.

Amen.

XXXXX

Be still in the presence of the Lord, and wait patiently for him to act. Don't worry about evil people who prosper or fret about their wicked schemes.

PSALM 37:7 NLT

BE STILL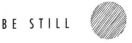

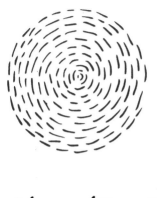

Chapter 3

GIVING AND RECEIVING

"Until now, you have asked nothing in My name.
Ask, and you will receive, that your joy may be full."

JOHN 16:24 NKJV

It had been only a few weeks since the collapse, and my health was deteriorating.

My doctors couldn't work out what was wrong or how to treat me. Fear was rife, and my hope waning.

Craig was out on the job; the kids were playing in the family room.

As I lay in the bubble bath, the mobile phone kept sounding messages in the next room.

Weak, disheartened by the lack of breakthrough, desperate for difference—for any improvement, I mumbled the occasional word prayer amidst the sobs.

Self-pity and physical weakness were my afternoon song that day. Feeling socially isolated and utterly alone, I burbled out a string of half words to God. "Send me something to show that You are here.

That You care. That it won't always be like this.

I need something to change."

Within minutes, I heard the sliding door open and then close.

A loud, friendly voice sounded.

Unable to respond, I just lay there.

There were words spoken with the kids, then footsteps. The bathroom door creaked open. The sense of defeat rendered me so weak that I couldn't lift my head to see who it was.

A friend, a beautifully loyal and loving friend, Lisa had arrived.

Gingerly, she walked in and found a complete mess, my face reddened and swollen from the tears and mucus.

She bent down and sat beside the bath.

Thankfully, I had some strategically placed bubbles in this soaking mess, but at this point, I simply didn't care.

Just seeing her, the slow but constant stream of tears became large fat drops pouring from my eyes. I cried and cried and cried. With its flow came release.

SHE LISTENED. SHE CARED. SHE DIDN'T GIVE ME ANY OPINIONS OR JUDGMENTS.

She listened. She cared. She didn't give me any opinions or judgments.

She listened some more and then prayed. It wasn't a long prayer. It was a prayer of support, authority, and love.

Lisa was like Moses' friends were to him (Exodus 17:12), lifting my arms for me when I couldn't, when I simply didn't have the strength.

Lifting them high, so the battle could be fought and won.

It was as though God was bringing me soothing tones of: ***"Don't give up.***

It won't always be like this.

You are not alone.

You're going to be okay."

There wasn't a miraculous change or anything immediate, but to know that God had answered my prayer was enough. Communicating to me that He was with me and cared. This was a priceless moment and gift to my heart.

God bless you, precious Lise.

As I journaled with God thinking about all the people investing in my family and me, since becoming unwell. It had been overwhelming.

DON'T GIVE UP. IT WON'T ALWAYS BE LIKE THIS.

A steady stream of people helping.

I slept through most of it.

Not only did I have consistent fear amidst a mystery illness, which rendered me physically useless. I was now freshly confronted by the kindness of others.

"God, I can't give anyone anything. I don't know what to do. I've always been able to give, and receiving is uncomfortable."

Family members, a handful of close friends, and strangers began helping our family. As I wrote a record of the people and things I could remember, the page was quickly filled.

Practical things. Taking the kids to school. Cleaning, cooking, prayer for my healing. They were faithful, loving people who wanted to help. They wanted to do something, anything.

It sometimes made me feel worse.

Watching their faces as they saw my depleted state. Unable to feign a smile or respond with my usual thankful heart.

GIVING AND RECEIVING

I saw faces of compassion, or was it pity?

My mind filled with thoughts about these people.

They are doing it because they are sorry for you.

You're a charity case.

You will never be able to pay them back.

Lord, it's too much. This is horrible. I feel helpless.

I didn't want others to know I couldn't do it.

I didn't want my weakness known.

This left me feeling even more debilitated than I was physically. As these capable men and women arrived at my door, bringing gifts of provision, it highlighted my own brokenness.

These people were the former me.

Who am I now if I can't do this for others anymore?

I feel like I owe them a debt, which I can never hope to repay.

They've been so kind to me—to us.

"What am I supposed to do with this, Lord?"

"It's your season to learn how to receive. You've been a good and faithful giver. Now it's time to learn how it feels for those you've been giving to."

My head instinctively bowed. Humbled as the truth of this statement landed deeply. I AM a terrible receiver in every aspect. I found gifts and attention in any form so hard to accept.

God, You know me so well.

"Every gift, every meal, every person bringing encouragement. I sent them. They are from Me, My child. Accept them as direct acts of love from Me."

Whoa....

It was difficult to accept from people, but how can I reject a gift directly from God?

Then it hit me.

These people are my village.

They are my church.

They are my community.

I tried to reason it all out.

Receiving is tough. Receiving is being vulnerable and open.

> IT WAS DIFFICULT TO ACCEPT FROM PEOPLE, BUT HOW CAN I REJECT A GIFT DIRECTLY FROM GOD?

Receiving commands a response, doesn't it? And I didn't quite know how to respond to all of this.

To remember all that my village had done for me.

To acknowledge all the time invested.

To thank all those who prayed with and for me.

To appreciate the few who stuck by me through thick and thin.

"How can I possibly hope to thank them? Lord, I feel overwhelmed, trying to remember all that they've done for me."

"These treasured ones don't help because they want thanks. They come, and they give because they want to help. This is what they know to

GIVING AND RECEIVING

do. By rejecting their help, for some, you reject them. By receiving their gift, you receive them."

Another challenging but essential truth, Lord.

I've rejected help so often in the past. I've felt the discomfort of "need."

I'm so sorry for those I've injured by being so self-reliant, Lord.

Please forgive me.

"You have permission to begin to receive well, My daughter. No lists. No one owes another. My heart is that you give AND receive in life. This is a time when others will pick you up. And when you have regained your strength, you will pick others up again.

This is village. This is My church in action. Receive. Receive. Receive."

Yes, God is more than ready to overwhelm you with every
form of grace so that you will have more than enough of
everything—every moment and in every way. He will make
you overflow with abundance in every good thing you do.

2 CORINTHIANS 9:8 TPT

The LORD is trustworthy in all he promises
and faithful in all he does.

The Lord upholds all who fall
and lifts up all who are bowed down.

The eyes of all look to you,
and you give them their food at the proper time.

You open your hand
and satisfy the desires of every living thing.

The Lord is righteous in all his ways
and faithful in all he does.

The Lord is near to all who call on him,
to all who call on him in truth.

PSALM 145:13B-18 NIV

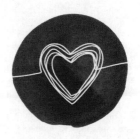

— Father's Heart —

*"Oh, My precious child, let Me lavish My
love upon you during this time.*

I have abundant supplies readily available for you.

*I have told you to ask anything in My name, and
you will receive that your joy may be full.*

Do you believe this, My child?

Will you choose to trust Me?

*I know that at times you've felt guilty
about receiving from others.*

*These ones I send bring you symbols of My
love, My attention, and care.*

*You are so special to Me; I have not forgotten you
and have much in store for you, My love.*

Just as you have poured into others, I desire to pour into you.

*Take heart, when you receive from ones
such as these, You receive from Me.*

When you welcome them in, you welcome Me in.

*As you feel the warmth that comes from being seen
and cared for in these ways, you accept Me.*

*You are My precious child; I want to
nurture you if you will allow Me.*

*Understand that I've made you to give and to
receive in life. Not one wholly or the other. But
seasons, moments of giving and receiving.*

Receiving in My kingdom is also to give.

To give to others is also to receive.

*To give and receive from a pure heart—
well, there is no greater gift.*

*I am the true giver and the One you will
receive from constantly. My desire is to be
abundantly generous to My children.*

This is lived out in relationship with Me.

But by receiving from others, you also receive from Me.

There is much in your life vying for your energy and time.

*Where will you choose to invest it? Will you
come alongside Me and commune?*

*I have kingdom adventures for you and me to unite in.
Never before will you experience such blessing than when
you have chosen to partner with the plans of My heart.*

My heart and yours in sweet embrace.

*My provision poured out, My words, My
acts of love…I have brought these and more
for you to be a part of, My beloved.*

GIVING AND RECEIVING

I invite you each day.

Come, let's adventure together, let's talk and walk a while,
and I will lift you to higher plains of giving and receiving."

Give, and it will be given to you: good measure,
pressed down, shaken together, and running over,
will be given to you. For with the same measure
you measure, it will be measured back to you.

LUKE 6:38 WEB

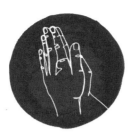

— *Prayer* —

Abundant, generous, and loving God,

Thank You for being the ultimate gift giver.

*It is humbling to receive from others
and from You at times, Lord.*

Please show me how to be gracious in my giving and receiving.

Let my response to receiving be to give thanks and glorify You.

Bless those who have given to me in this season.

Thank You for their kindness and love.

*Show me how to step into Your river of
life-giving flow. As the need arises and You've given
me resource, let it flow out to fulfill that need.*

*As I ask You for what I need, let me keep watch
for how You will meet that need... Thank You for
Your dependable promises to be my provider.*

Jehovah Jirah, I trust You.

Amen.

XXXXX

GIVING AND RECEIVING

All generous giving and every perfect gift is from above,
coming down from the Father of lights, with whom
there is no variation or the slightest hint of change.

JAMES 1:17 NET

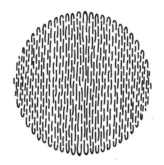

Chapter 4

ATMOSPHERE

And He said, "My Presence will go with
you, and I will give you rest."

EXODUS 33:14 NKJV

We'd just moved into our new house. Winter was fast approaching. As the temperature cooled, we noticed just how dark and chilly our new abode was. Having been afflicted for most of my time in this home, the atmosphere seemed to reflect my health status. After recognizing the impact the lack of natural light inside was having on me, I began talking to God about it.

Lord, this home is so dark and cold. I can't get outside or drive to escape. I need something to change. My healing seems to have stalled with living in this place.

He responded in three ways in a short space of time.

The first of our atmosphere changes began one intense week.

I'd been struggling with sleepless nights and sent out a prayer request for help to my prayer warrior friends.

"Ding ding!" my phone chimed the following morning. A beautiful friend, Wendy, had messaged, wanting to drop something in. It turned out it was the Bethel, "Be Lifted High" CD. I'd never heard of Bethel or their album but was open to anything at this point. She'd been given a gentle prompt the previous night to drop it in.

That afternoon, I laid out on my couch and listened to the heavenly sounds.

The fear that had been my constant since the moment I collapsed, dissipated.

The nervous energy was replaced with His peace.

For the first time in months, I found myself feeling relaxed and less "wired."

> **I PLACED THE MUSIC ON REPEAT AND LET IT SOAK INTO EVERY CELL OF MY BODY.**

I placed the music on repeat and let it soak into every cell of my body. I barely noticed as the hours ticked by. The parched land of my heart drank in the wellspring of life. The lyrics spoke to the atmosphere of my heart, and as it turns out, our home.

My ears absorbed the sweetness of the sound, and my body responded positively.

In this time of soaking God gently prompted.

"What do you tell your children?"

I knew instinctively what He was talking about.

I had always told our kids that whatever you allow your eyes and ears to see and hear goes into your mind. These can be for your good or not.

Images of what I'd been watching, listening to, and inadvertently been absorbing flooded into my mind.

What was I allowing my senses to encounter?

Desperate for something relational and "normal," I'd watched every DVD we had, listened to the radio, and generally kept connected to the world.

A lightbulb moment!

They weren't bad things in themselves, but they weren't healthy for me in this season.

I felt another idea come in loud and clear.

"Take a sabbatical from everything that takes from you, fill your day with all that is life-giving."

Only God could give me permission to do this, and a sense of great anticipation stirred within me as I pondered what might result.

The very next morning, I turned off the radio, TV, and all other technology. If it didn't bring positive or uplifting messages, I didn't want to engage with it.

I went outside into the sunshine, listening to worship music most of the time.

I signed up for various Bible verse apps and only read and listened to what would feed the seedling of hope within my heart.

I noted over the week, the spiritual atmosphere of our home was transformed. I felt lighter and more hopeful. There was a greater sense of peace and order in our home. Fear was now an irregular intruder rather than a constant prowler.

Thank You, Lord!

After this miraculous change, God healed the second aspect of our home atmosphere.

Being in the center of our lightless home, our kitchen was dark. To cut, clean, or cook, we relied upon a lone bulb. It was challenging for my light-loving heart. I began to talk to God about the light. Or maybe it was to air my complaints to Him about the light.

I noticed a few strange things began to happen.

ATMOSPHERE

The first was that our letterbox regularly began receiving pamphlets for skylights and special discounted prices for installing skylights.

The second was Bible verse apps began sending daily verses, which were all focused upon the theme of light.

The third happened as I watched late night/early morning sermons on television. I began seeing skylight advertisements—something I had never seen or noticed before. It all seemed "random"—independent of one another but put together over a few weeks, and it felt like a God setup.

"What does this all mean?"

Becoming more aware of messages and signs from God was a new thing for me, but He had made it so apparent to me that something was going on.

I sensed Him reply, *"Time to get a skylight quote."*

So I did.

I picked up one from the pile of pamphlets we'd discovered in our letterbox and called.

The special discounted price proved very reasonable, but I struggled internally about the cost. Financially, we had been living week to week. It was a season of financial faith walking. To spend money on a nonessential item seemed extravagant. We mutually decided to wait on God.

Miraculously, an unexpected windfall appeared in our bank account for a little more than the cost of the quote we'd received that same week. We took this as a sign to go ahead with the installation.

My heart flew to such high heights, as for the first time in our new home, I could see our kitchen bench without turning on a lightbulb. I found myself in awe of how a small gift can bring such life!

For this is what the LORD says—he who created the heavens, he is God, He who fashioned and made the earth, he founded it; He did not create it to be empty, but formed it to be inhabited—he says; "I am the LORD, and there is no other."

ISAIAH 45:18 NIV

Thank You, God!

A month or so following this event, our home atmosphere upgrade's third and final installment occurred.

The temperature was dropping, and sadly our sole source of heat began behaving strangely. As our home had no insulation and the timber flooring was laid directly over the dirt floor beneath, the earth's cool seemed to radiate upward, making our home not unlike an icebox.

One particular morning I tried turning on the heater.

Click…click…odd clanking sounds…a strange smell…that's new.

The delays and sounds had been happening for weeks, but the smell…. Something was definitely wrong.

"Call the repairman." A gentle prompt.

That sounds wise.

Walking around like a nomadic tent dweller with every piece of winter clothing on my body, I made the call.

Thankfully, he could check our system the very next day.

The doorbell rang, and I met Greg, a 20-year veteran in heating and air conditioning building and repair. After chatting for a while, I took him out to see our system. Then swiftly headed back inside to stand in front of the electric oven to keep warm.

Greg wasn't there for long.

He came to the back door, face ashen. He explained that our system was broken.

"You are all lucky to be alive!" he articulated. Explaining the intricacies of the silent killer, I tried to take in what he was saying, but all I heard was *gas, people dying as they slept, can't smell it.*

I was in shock.

Then a revelation and strong sense of God's protection increased. My heart became increasingly thankful instead of pondering the what-ifs. This, too, was a miracle.

Greg replaced the broken part, and we enjoyed two months of blissful heating.

Unfortunately, after two months of heated heaven, the same strange sound returned.

Greg swiftly returned and found that the broken piece was again broken. "I've not seen anything like this in 20 years."

It had an eerie feeling about it, even for this down-to-earth, practical fella. "It might be a good idea to get rid of this system; there's something weird about it."

"YOU ARE ALL LUCKY TO BE ALIVE!" HE ARTICULATED.

"How much is a new one?" I inquired, knowing full well we didn't have much of anything financially.

"It varies, but for a house like yours, you are looking at about $1800."

My jaw dropped at the price, knowing this was humanly unattainable for us. I fought back the tears. The cold definitely exacerbated my symptoms, and we could not afford a new heater.

What now, Lord?

I found myself explaining to Greg our situation. "We just don't have the money. Since becoming unwell, I've not been able to work, and my hubby has been taking care of me. I don't know how we're going to do this, Greg."

I saw a look of compassion and understanding come over Greg's face as he explained how his family had gone through some tough

ATMOSPHERE

times recently as well. He then poured out his own family's health challenge story, and this tough Australian guy teared up a little as he shared. What a privilege to listen to him in his pain!

Shared weakness opened up an opportunity for encouragement.

It struck me as strange that God would use my pain to help with his.

It was at this moment that Greg had an aha moment!

Remembering, he had a one-year-old system sitting in his garage at home, he told me that he'd been called out on a job to remove it because it was too hot for the older owners. I stood there again with my mouth open and shaking my head in amazement.

Tears of joy began stirring within my depths and bubbling up. God had gone ahead of this whole situation. I waited, wondering what would happen next.

SHARED WEAKNESS
OPENED UP AN
OPPORTUNITY FOR
ENCOURAGEMENT.

"You can have it for $150 and install time if you like." He was apologetic about charging me anything, but he'd have to buy some parts to fit it for us.

I couldn't believe it! God had provided for us again in an extraordinary way.

I leaped with glee inside and profusely thanked Greg for his kindness.

I could tell that he couldn't believe what had happened either, saying, "I never got why they'd get rid of a heater for being too hot."

As Greg left, the journey of our dysfunctional system that almost gassed us twice hit home.

Thank You, God! Thank You, God!

I've no words to express the relief I feel that You protected us all. And now You've provided a way out in an incredible way. How does this happen, Lord?"

It was now being exchanged with a nearly new system. Only God could orchestrate this upgrade. The following day Greg returned to replace our old with the new. I'd never been so happy to see the back of something or so delighted about an appliance being installed. Melbourne winter had never looked so good.

God had taken the dark, cold, and health-crushing atmosphere of our house, turning it for my good into a light-filled, warm place of spiritual blessing.

"God, You made our house into a home."

Over the following year, I began to experience improvement in my health due to all that God had done in this time.

ATMOSPHERE

— Father's Heart —

"I am the King of all environments. No atmosphere or situation is greater than I am.

As I live in you, you take My presence wherever you go. As you become more conscious of our journeying together, I will equip you with everything you need.

When an atmosphere is heavy and burdening, bring Me into your situation, and there will be shift.

Acknowledge and trust Me wherever you find yourself.

I am tangible and real. Although you don't often see My form with your eyes, I am more real than anything you might see.

The spirit realm is continually moving, as do I.

I never sleep. As you become aware of Me, you will experience what happens when I come into a situation. The weight of heaviness is shared between us both.

I love nothing better than to carry the bulk. Bringing redemptive elements for you in what remains.

Cast your heaviness on Me. My Son died so you don't have to live under burdens anymore.

*Flow with My Spirit. He will lift the air
around you just because you are there, and
He lives within it and within you.*

*Oppressive atmospheres, negativity, or lack?
These are My kinds of spaces, which I love
to infiltrate and redeem through you.*

What can stand against you as I dwell in you? Nothing.

Do you have opposition, fear, upset, anxiety, or grief?

*Let Me shift that for you. Let Me exchange
the atmosphere for My truth.*

*Let Me inject My peace, My love, My
comfort, My embrace into your situation.*

*I do not do this so that you might be comfortable, but
that we would commune with one another. And that you
might share with others the reason for your joy and hope.*

*That you would be a temple for My Holy Spirit, and that
temple is brought into the world to change the world.*

In Me, you are a true world changer.

Start small if you are unsure; I don't mind small beginnings.

*Those small steps of trust lead to greater confidence
in My ability to work-whatever comes your way.*

*Nothing stands in the way of My ability to
change atmospheres and circumstances."*

ATMOSPHERE

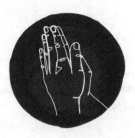

— Prayer —

Precious Father, Holy Spirit, and Jesus,

Our home and everything we have is Yours. Let these
things never take the place of You in our hearts.

Please flush out anything that doesn't belong.
Let Your Holy Spirit abide and be evident
in our home, in Jesus' powerful name.

Please show me how to enhance the atmosphere
around me so that Your presence feels welcome.

For where You are, there too is Your fruit.

Love, joy, peace, patience, kindness, goodness,
faithfulness, and self-control...I desire these
for our home and family atmosphere.

Keep my heart soft to the things of You, Father, and
to the sound of Your tender voice as You guide,
encourage, and provide a way for home to be a haven.

You know, in tough times, this is
essential for health and for hope.

I am so thankful for this key of change
being brought into my life.

Thank You for caring about every aspect of life.

You are such a good, good God.

Amen.

XXXXX

They traded the truth about God for a lie.
So they worshipped and served the things God
created instead of the Creator himself, who
is worthy of eternal praise! Amen.

ROMANS 1:25 NLT

ATMOSPHERE

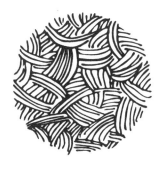

Chapter 5

NEVER ALONE

The one who sent me is with me; he has not left
me alone, for I always do what pleases Him.

JOHN 8:29 NIV

Standing at my kitchen bench, gazing off into the distance, my thoughts raced.

This morning had been another fruitless doctor's appointment. Disappointment, disillusionment, and frustration were rife as I let all that had happened land within me.

Where is my healing? Where are the answers? I feel so alone in all of this.

"You are not alone; I am with you," His tender voice whispered in response.

My heart—tired of carrying it all and not having a single person who could relate to my mystery illness. No one who could humanly toss me a sliver of hope or answer.

I felt frustrated by mainstream medical answers, "…eat a high salt diet, drink water, and rest." *I've been doing this for months.*

As I pondered whether life was ever going to get any better, I fought off the seeds of hopelessness, which endeavored to take root in me.

"Turn to Me," a gentle whisper came.

I wasn't in the mood to listen right now. I wanted action and change.

Without warning, my head suddenly Whooooooosssssshhhhed. "Oh, no!"

The room began to spin, and my eyes instinctively shut tight. Grabbing hold of the edge of the bench, I steadied my unbalanced body, which was desperate to fall to the floor.

I awkwardly made my way towards the nearby kitchen chair. Plomping heavily down into it, I laid my head on the tabletop and allowed the world to stop spinning. Hoping that the spinning inside my brain might cease as I rested somewhere firm and flat.

The last time this had happened, I'd been shopping at a stationery store. The air conditioner had been blowing hard as I'd walked through the front doors, creating an icy brain sensation. I'd made it to the computer section, and then down, down, down I went. I lay there as song after song played in the background; no one came. Customers buzzed past; an employee even stepped over my head. It was as if I was invisible. I was alone. It was then that the tears began to flow, just as they were now.

Let's try positive self-talk, Karen.

This is different. You are at home. You need to be present in this moment— not back there. This isn't the same. Forget the worry. Forget the past experiences. Connect with God? Connect with God!

He always makes me feel better.

This thought disappeared as quickly as it came in, as fear butted its unhelpful head in.

I need someone's help, and no one is home. What do I do? I'm scared.

This pain. This dizziness. Help!

"Look how far you've come, beloved," He lovingly reassured and comforted me.

It's true. I have come a long way. I am not the lump of exhausted jelly spread out on the couch anymore. I can stand. I can walk, albeit slowly. I can track ideas better than before. Things are definitely on the improve.

"But where is my 'living life to the full,' Jesus?"

"BUT WHERE IS MY 'LIVING LIFE TO THE FULL,' JESUS?"

It felt as if I was imprisoned—an isolating prison of measured living.

Time ticked by. How long? I never can tell.

"Don't think. Don't stress. Don't ponder too much. Don't look back.

Just be."

Without warning, a pang of fear zapped in. Everything escalated as the fear quickly snowballed into an avalanche of ideas and thoughts.

I'm tired of the battle.

Fear led to sorrow, which met discouragement. Giant salty sobs trekked their way down my cheeks, across my nose, dripping onto the table.

In the kitchen, the tap drips as if to mirror my sadness: so many symptoms, so much mystery. Every time I went to the doctor, it was for the symptomatic rather than the core issue.

No one seems to understand it all. Lord, I feel so alone in this—even with those who care surrounding me. I am so alone; no one "gets it."

The sun went behind a cloud.

My head has stopped whooshing, the world has stopped spinning, my heart isn't racing. Maybe I can resume an upright position? Time to get back to the rest of those dishes.

NEVER ALONE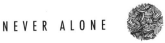

As I moved, I began pondering my brilliant, God-given medical team, my faithful alternative therapy GP, naturopath, and chiropractor. They'd gotten me upright and moving once again when mainstream medicine shrugged their shoulders, unsure of any next step. "Perhaps it's all in your head," they'd suggested.

What a devastating blow it had been today! They had nothing more to offer me; I'd come to the end of the mainstream line.

There had been so many specialists, tests, appointments, and racing about—an ongoing search, desperate to find THE answer, desperate for complete healing, not just band-aids.

> WHEN THE WORLD HAS NOTHING MORE TO OFFER, IT IS A PROFOUNDLY TERRIFYING AND STRANGELY FREEING MOMENT.

When I asked, God hadn't told me to race. He'd told me my healing would come in the still. But humanly, I couldn't just leave it and do nothing. Could I?

I was tired of waiting. I would find my own cure through others.

There must be an answer out there somewhere. He loved me through my choice to push on. To turn to others.

"This isn't the end for you, child. I am with you. I love you."

Now the tears became like Niagara Falls of flow. Self-pity seemed to be reigning at this moment.

A deep sadness as the realization, "I have come to the end of myself." No more ability to come up with answers. No control over my future or over my health. Nothing more to bring. Mainstream doctors seem to have nothing else to offer me. Nothing. Humanly, I feel alone in this.

When the world has nothing more to offer, it is a profoundly terrifying and strangely freeing moment.

I'd been through many tough times as a believer, but this was on a whole other level. The faith that I'd held so dear for decades. I needed to actually walk out the trust element, like never before.

I have no other choice but to wholly trust God. Because the only other option is to live without hope. And that, to me, is not a viable alternative.

Standing at the end of my burgundy benchtop. I pulled the plug to let out the now cool water.

I HAVE NO OTHER CHOICE BUT TO WHOLLY TRUST GOD. BECAUSE THE ONLY OTHER OPTION IS TO LIVE WITHOUT HOPE. AND THAT, TO ME, IS NOT A VIABLE ALTERNATIVE.

As the water pooled at the bottom of the sink and headed down the drainpipe. Before me, a fresh, clean sink.

Ready to begin again?

What do I do now?

Something was stirring within me.

Strength? Fresh resolve!

I tossed my hands up in the air, and with deep abandon, cried out to God.

"Father, I don't know what is happening. Whether I will die suddenly or live for decades to come. I don't want to be fearful, but I need something. I need Your help."

At that very moment, something "random" popped in unexpectedly.

NEVER ALONE

And I am convinced that nothing can ever separate
us from God's love. Neither death nor life, neither
angels nor demons, neither our fears for today nor
our worries about tomorrow-not even the powers of
hell can separate us from God's love. NO power in the
sky above or in the earth below-indeed, nothing in all
of creation will ever be able to separate us from the
love of God that is revealed in Christ Jesus our Lord.

ROMANS 8:38-39 NLT

A thought. A quiet revelation.

"I have been putting out spot fires of symptoms rather than dealing with the raging blaze of affliction. No mainstream doctor had heard the whole story from start to finish." *What an idea!*

I was taken aback. The tears eased off, and a laugh bubbled up as I pondered this light-bulb moment.

Relief had pierced the tension—a release of pressure—the power of some laughter. Realizing that this could be the way forward.

"God, was that You?"

Before He could respond, I chimed in, "Of course, it was. Who else could come up with such a revolutionary plan?!"

A stirring began to whip about, building hope-filled anticipation in my heart.

Then before I knew it, something happened that I have not experienced before or since. In my mind's eye, God began typing letters before me.

One letter at a time—as if they were actually being typed by the Father on a vintage typewriter.

The letters were typed in goldfields poster font. Spelling the name of a local general practitioner. My mouth agape, I stood in sheer awe of what God was doing before me. Rendering me speechless. I dared not move as this was too amazing, and I didn't want it to end.

The possibilities of what this could mean struck me, and I found myself unable to stop praising Him.

"God, You are incredible! Thank You. Thank You. Thank You."

Beyond excited and so touched that Father would speak to me in such a personal way. Knowing that I love typewriters, vintage elements,

NEVER ALONE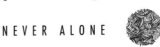

> I DARED NOT
> MOVE AS THIS
> WAS TOO
> AMAZING, AND
> I DIDN'T WANT
> IT TO END.

the goldfields, and everything letters, type fonts, and language.

Everything was designed to communicate, "I see you, I know you, I love you personally." The tears continued to flow, but they rushed for a different reason this time—for joy.

God saw what was happening. God heard my cries. He cared. I am not alone because He is with me. That very afternoon I made an appointment with Dr. Tania.

One week later, as I sat in her office, I let it all out—from start to finish. Complete transparency. No detail left unsaid.

She patiently listened, occasionally nodding.

As I finished up, the energy in the room was palpable.

She looked at me from behind her gold-rimmed glasses. She gently leaned on the arm of her chair as she shifted. Touching the arm of her glasses, she carefully considered all that I had communicated.

The regular migraine diagnosis was suggested but was then quickly discounted.

The tears began to flow once again. I pressed in. Explaining that God had given me her name, so she must know the next step in my healing journey.

I was pretty messy at this point. Tears, mucus, and the like, but I was also beyond caring what others thought of me. As I released that statement of truth to her, a boldness came over me. This uncharacteristic boldness reassured me that Holy Spirit was in me and in this situation.

The atmosphere in the room exchanged its nervous fear for peace. I knew without a shadow of a doubt that God was with me in that room. I was determined to remain until He communicated what He brought me here for.

We both sat in silence, me in bold peace, and she, processing mode. I noticed that her eyes began to glisten a little. Like the beginnings of an idea was coming to mind. And in a moment, I knew she had it.

She quietly spoke out the name of a diagnostic specialist who was not unlike the doctor from the television series, *House*. He was a specialist across three fields and was someone who seemed to have great insight into difficult cases, like mine.

Dr. Tania grinned from ear to ear, and we celebrated a little together at this "random" idea that had popped into her mind. She was pleased to print me a referral, and as I headed out of her office, my heart felt light and full of hope once again.

It was the first time in eighteen months I had relied entirely on God—not on myself or others. He had lovingly tended to me in my tears, partnering with me in formulating and executing a plan. And answered me in more brilliant ways than I could have ever hoped for. And it felt great!

— Father's Heart —

*"How can I communicate to you more
strongly about how much I love you?*

*I tell you that you are never alone, yet you don't always
feel it, you don't always see it, and doubt can creep in.*

Trust Me, My precious child.

*I created you before the beginning of time. My mind
knew the inner workings of your entire being. I
knew how you would live, what your personality
would be. I even knew the special moments we would
share throughout your lifetime here on earth.*

All of this, well before you were born.

*I have created you from dust, someone so entirely precious
to Me from something that seems relatively worthless.*

*If you understood the value I place upon you, you
would never question whether or not you were
alone. That you are alone is simply a lie.*

*My truth is that you are very much known,
and I am your constant companion.*

I love you, My child.

*You are remembered every second of the
day and night. I love you, My child.*

*You have no idea how many thoughts I have
about you. They outnumber the grains of
sand on all the beaches of the world.*

You are so special to Me.

You hold such great worth and importance to Me.

*I know there have been times when you felt
worthless and unimportant; that too is a lie.*

*I exist, and I cover everything. My Spirit moves over the
earth, and My heavenly beings and I watch over you.*

*I am fully aware of what you are feeling
right at this moment…and I care.*

*I am not absent or far away, as you sometimes feel, but
I am closer than your breath. I love you that much.*

My beloved, when you feel isolated, come to Me.

Decide to wait with Me and upon Me.

*Ask Me to reveal Myself to you, and I
will fill the empty space.*

*I will do this because it is who I am, and it is
what I LOVE to do—especially for you."*

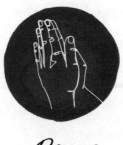

— Prayer —

Father, there are times when I have felt alone.

*But when I come to you, I begin to see
how You've been so near, so constant.*

*As I speak all that fills my mind, You
whisper words of life to me.*

*Verses read long ago come to my
heart and begin to settle me.*

*You encourage me that I am never alone, for
You are always with me (Matthew 28:20b).*

*You reassure me that you have gone ahead of me
and walk beside me whatever I am going through
(Deuteronomy 31:8), This comforts me in the tough.*

*Thank You for Your truth that I am never alone, and
I am never forgotten. There is always hope in You.*

I choose to trust You today with my situation.

*With Your help, I will not allow
this to be bigger than You.*

*Please guide me as I walk forward in Your
strength, knowing You are with me.*

*When I am with You and You are with
me, there is no other place I want to be.*

Amen.

✗✗✗✗✗

Don't be afraid, for I am with you.
Don't be discouraged, for I am your God.
I will strengthen you and help you.
I will hold you up with my victorious right hand.

ISAIAH 41:10 NLT

NEVER ALONE

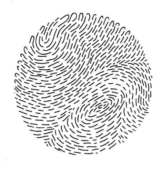

Chapter 6

SAFE PLACES AND SAFE PEOPLE

Do to others as you would have them do to you.

LUKE 6:31 NIV

Today was a hard day.

I was confused. There were so many opinions, ideas on how I could be healed.

I'd run everywhere to try and find my healing, all to no avail.

As I journaled out this heavy day with God, I began writing down my jumbled thoughts and questions. I poured out the words of some, and as I did, I could freshly hear their voices.

"Maybe you've got an unconfessed sin that you don't know about."

"You have a spirit of affliction in you."

"Have you prayed enough?"

"Have you been to a deliverance ministry?"

"You must have a demon in you."

"Maybe there is someone you haven't forgiven."

"God says if you have faith as small as a mustard seed, have you considered your faith isn't big enough."

My body and mind groaned as each one spoken to me at my most vulnerable added fuel to the fire. The fire which preached at me, "There's no way out. You aren't doing enough. It's going to get worse. There's no hope."

Some days I drew the few remaining drops from my tank to broach these possibilities—each one leading me to dry wastelands.

WHAT IF MY FAITH ISN'T BIG ENOUGH?

I had tried to raise each one with God... but they came so thick and fast, and I barely had enough energy to get out of bed, let alone give processing space for these words to be weighed and measured.

And yet, they did land. All these throwaway comments served to do was to pile more upon my weary frame. As the doubts and fears rolled over in waves in my mind. I endeavored to evaluate each one, desperate for an answer.

What if my faith isn't big enough?

How can I do more when I can barely do the basics?

How do I work out if I haven't forgiven someone?

I'd forgive them if I knew? Wouldn't God remind me? What if I was supposed to work it all out by myself? What if it is demonic? What do I believe about deliverance and the demonic?

Images of the little I knew of the demon side of things rattled around my mind, which put me straight into a terrified mode.

I had no idea what to do. I'd not encountered some of these areas in decades of faith. Now seemed the worst possible time to try and get to the bottom of belief.

These overwhelming possibilities ensured anxiety and fear were well-fed.

My inner perfectionist entertained them, giving them pride of place.

I know this is no way to live, but how do I come to peace, Father, with things I'm unsure of? Why is this happening to me? Did I do something?

Am I being punished for something? Is my body paying me back for the years of neglect? What if any of these people's words are right?

Unhelpful words from good, well-intentioned people.

Each time I spoke with someone, my thoughts began to have a knee-jerk reaction as I internally questioned their safety. Their intent. *What will come out of their mouth next?* Unfortunately, a sprinkling of unsafe people tainted the rest at this time.

Am I safe with them? Can I be honest with them? Will they hurt me?

These people wanted my healing as much as I did. I could see and feel that. They wanted my best. It was confronting to see their beloved friend in pain. A shadow of her former self, unable to be who she once was. Loving people struggling with their own theologies of healing, wrestling with why God wasn't healing me in the way we all hoped for and expected.

I could tangibly see them reasoning it out. "God is good. Karen isn't healed; there MUST be a reason why. She has done something. Or hasn't done something? Or could or should do something?"

Some continued to bring "answers, reasons, and explanations as to why it might not have come."

I couldn't help them with their questions. I had the same ones.

Each time, my heart was left a little more bruised—a little more battered as I sank beneath the waves.

SAFE PLACES AND SAFE PEOPLE

You are my hiding place. You will protect me from
trouble and surround me with songs of deliverance.

PSALM 32:7 NIV

Living with this affliction was burden enough.

Lord, why are some loading more on me? And more importantly, why am I letting them?

As I journaled with God on this hard day, He reminded me of the verse He had given me many times before: Luke 11:46. "Jesus replied, 'And you experts in the law, woe to you, because you load people down with burdens they can hardly carry, and you yourselves will not lift one finger to help them.'"

This burden of others expectations, unmet hopes and prayers, weighed heavily upon my heart.

I hated seeing the look of disappointment come across their faces when prayers seemed to go unheard and unanswered. They were weary from the intensity, the lack of breakthrough all these past months.

It was gut wrenching to watch me experience pain, and waves of mysterious symptoms-all of which stole the woman they once knew-seemingly without purpose.

For some, I wasn't who they wanted or needed me to be.

Confused, I shared my exposed heart with God.

What am I supposed to do with this, Lord? I feel like I don't know who to listen to anymore.

The world is a harsh place for me. I have nowhere to go for help. What am I to do?

My heart cried out, "I need safety, Lord!"

"Call the church office."

Hesitantly, I obeyed the gentle, sweet whisper and rang. God had gone ahead of my call. A kind male voice answered; it was Pastor Ken.

SAFE PLACES AND SAFE PEOPLE

Surely it was unusual to have the lead pastor answer the phone at reception?

I was thankful—one less conversation to have. Relieved, I nestled back into the comfy couch, ready to ask some BIG questions. Feeling the tiniest seed of hope that God had a reason for prompting the call.

OH, MY HEART. I SEE YOU. I REMEMBER YOUR SOFTNESS. I'M SO THANKFUL THAT YOU CAN BE SAFE HERE.

I held it together, not wanting to download everything in one big lump and overwhelm the poor man.

"Hi, Ken," I said as chipperly as I could muster.

"Oh, g'day, Karen. How are you going?" he responded.

Hearing his kind voice. Having someone ask sincerely how I was going without agenda or ulterior motive, I was immediately undone.

My heart let down its protective shell. The pieces I'd haphazardly nailed up fell away—one part at a time. Like pieces of armor, they dropped off, recognizing instantly that there was no threat here today.

Oh, my heart. I see you. I remember your softness. I'm so thankful that you can be safe here.

I welled up and then blinked. The tears dribbled from the corners of my eyes, and again I was amazed at how much can happen in a split second when safe.

"This feels safe. I am safe. My heart can be itself here."

Thank You, Lord.

"What's going on?" Ken asked gently.

And like my salty tears, everything poured out.

I shared with him the things that I felt. I spoke about the words people had put out into my already stretched brain and the weightiness which was pulling heavily upon my heart. I shared about the internal conflict I felt and how fearful and confused I was about it all.

He patiently listened, giving a reassuring mmm..mmmm....sound every so often to let me know he was still listening.

How wonderful is it to have someone just listen. Thank You, God.

I shared with him how I had run here and there, hoping to be healed. Trusting, I'd be healed...believing I'd be healed.

I told him about the well-meaning people sharing their well-intentioned words. Words that, instead of freedom, had left me feeling condemned. It was more burden than I had the capacity for.

Ken listened and didn't interrupt or offer justifications or opinions of his own. He just heard my heart, intently and lovingly.

Sharing with Ken felt like how I communicated with Jesus. I was safe, sheltered, and secure. There was nothing to fear here.

The tears lessened. Sharing openly with Ken was helping to lift the weight.

Having someone simply be present in my pain was the most valuable gift anyone could bring—someone to listen, to fully engage with what I was communicating. No judgment. No answers. Nothing but a caring heart and a listening ear.

When I had finally finished, with everything shared, I held my breath— not knowing but hoping that Ken would continue to be a safe place for my heart. Seconds passed; they felt like minutes.

Ken spoke.

SAFE PLACES AND SAFE PEOPLE

And as he spoke, it seemed they were the very words of Holy Spirit to me.

These were the words I had longed to hear. They felt like home.

> HAVING SOMEONE SIMPLY BE PRESENT IN MY PAIN WAS THE MOST VALUABLE GIFT ANYONE COULD BRING— SOMEONE TO LISTEN, TO FULLY ENGAGE WITH WHAT I WAS COMMUNICATING. NO JUDGMENT. NO ANSWERS. NOTHING BUT A CARING HEART AND A LISTENING EAR.

My heart relaxed. My mind felt as if balm was being applied. My spirit was given the clarity I'd hoped for.

He spoke words of truth. They were Father's words.

They came from a place of wanting to give me sound hope. Even when there was so much to contend with, there WAS hope.

Ken validated my heart.

He didn't try and explain all that was happening or justify the responses of others. He went to a higher, more beautiful place.

He explained how Father God doesn't want to load me down with heavy loads. He would never bring anything to cause me to fear.

He longs to bring me His peace because I am precious to Him.

I breathed in deeply, exhaling all the stress of these past few months.

What a gift this time has been.

Ken continued…"Karen, the Lord has brought to my mind this little verse. And I think it might help you, as it's helped me many times before."

He shared Romans 8:15 with me. "For you did not receive a spirit that makes you a slave to fear, but you received the Spirit of sonship. And by Him, we cry, 'Abba, Father.'"

He explained that this verse reassures me that I am a child of God, adopted by Him, and He has given me, as His child, a right to live free from fear—free from anything that holds me back. Anything that keeps me from freedom and peace. God was going to give me what I needed when I needed it.

My role was to receive what He was giving.

I didn't need to work it all out; I simply needed to let His voice be the one I listened to first and foremost. This truth-filled verse aligned my heart, mind, and questions with the Father's true nature. *He is my safe place.* When I have this truth before me, the words of others were put in their rightful place.

This day, this conversation, the kindness and "Father-heartedness" of Ken healed so much in me, and I'll be forever grateful.

Strengthened and with fresh clarity, I moved forward into the rest of the day. Having had so much put into perspective, my heart was light and free. Having been significantly encouraged by someone who proved himself a very safe person in a most significant moment.

— Father's Heart —

"I have placed My Holy Spirit within you. Part of His ways are to show you the truth about all things.

It is essential to know My heart for you is for your good.

When you accept this truth, it becomes much easier to discern the best way forward—with Me.

I am your safe place.

I have placed people around you who, like you, have needs and desires. Some of those needs and desires are healthy, and others are not.

My heart is that my children would live together in love, encouraging, considering, and serving one another. Giving grace and forgiveness where and when needed.

You are always safe with Me, beloved, but not all people and places are safe all the time. My desire is that you would have connection with safe people. Understand that no one person is wholly secure all the time. This is because all people are on their own journey through life and growth.

As you place Me at the forefront, you will experience complete safety in love. By encountering Me in this way, you will see aspects of Me in others.

As you connect with others, you may experience disappointment or hurt.

Take heart…with Me as your foundation, you will become accustomed to what safe places and people look and feel like.

Ask My Spirit for guidance as He won't lead you astray.

I will never bring fear or confusion. These things are not a part of My heart.

Know Me, and you will recognize what is or isn't My best for you.

Not all people have you in mind as they speak or act; they too are mid-process.

Forgive, My child. Forgive and bless those who have brought anything other than life to you. If their words or actions are in direct opposition to My words, then release them; don't hold onto these things. They are burdens you don't need to carry.

You have permission to weigh up others' words with Me. Let Me reveal My truth to you, precious one.

Rest assured, I have designed you to have healthy boundaries. I only ask of you what I have resourced and prepared you for.

Saying yes to all things and all people is never the way forward. I want you to say yes to the things and people I discern for you.

SAFE PLACES AND SAFE PEOPLE

*Place your expectations and needs at My feet and watch
how I bring the right people at the right times to you.*

*I know your heart longs to connect with healthy people
and be in safe relationship. I have designed you for
village life with others. Understand that the only wholly
complete friendship is Mine. Once you welcome this
truth, relationships with others will be healthier.*

*You have believed that to care for those in
community, you must be self-sacrificing. I never
asked you to be the sacrifice—only to bring others
to the One who was the sacrifice for them.*

*Love others wholeheartedly as I lead you, give them
grace in their own growth, and you will find they
will leave more deposits than withdrawals.*

Hold Me tightly and hold others lightly, beloved one.

You now know the way; follow it."

It is better to take refuge in the LORD
than to trust in humans.

PSALM 118:8 NIV

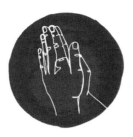

— *Prayer* —

To my ever-present safe place, Father God,

*Thank You that Your Presence is a
sweet and safe place to abide.*

*Guard my heart, Father, that I can be vulnerable
in safe relationship with those You bring to me, yet
still protected and led by Your Holy Spirit.*

*Please bring the right people at the right time along
this journey and speak words of life between us.*

Be at the center of all relationships, Lord God.

*Thank You for providing safe spaces that
minister to me in tough times.*

Thank You for being my ultimate provider and protector.

*Thank You for being my hiding place, protecting
me from trouble, and surrounding me with
songs of deliverance (Psalm 32:7).*

*Today I choose to trust You with this
area of safety, my loving God.*

Amen.

XXXXX

SAFE PLACES AND SAFE PEOPLE

Chapter 7

TRUST

I will save you; you will not fall by the
sword, but will escape with your life, Because
you trust in me, declares the LORD.

JEREMIAH 39:18 NIV

Laying there in my underwear in the middle of winter, waves of nausea washed over me. My heart raced like an internal setting switched to high—without the ability to turn it down.

When is this intensity going to stop rising?

It had been a massive day of cooking, cleaning, and resting. As with most productive days, I crashed towards the end, and this day was no exception.

Dinner was on the table, and after giving three dinner calls, I could feel my blood pressure dropping.

Glancing down at my feet, I likened them to elephant pads—full of fluid.

That's new.

I hadn't eaten in a few hours, and my body alerted me to that fact. I knew it needed something quicksmart, or I'd end up on the floor again.

I took a few mouthfuls just to carry me through, while the family s l o w l y made their way to the table.

Sitting there, my shoulders drooped as energy seemed to leak out of me. My stomach swirled, unhappy with the timing of what I'd given it. I'd left it too long. The familiar robust, sharp stabbing pains in my head returned as I tried not to cry at the intensity.

I carefully stood and went off to bed, not wanting the kids to see me swirl and sway.

The intensity began to rise, which mirrored my heart rate and pulse.

I wasn't anxious. I wasn't panicked. I was internally settled, but my heart rate just kept on rising.

> A DISTINCT DIFFERENCE ROSE UP FROM WITHIN— FRESH RESOLVE TO DO THIS TIME, DIFFERENTLY

As I rested on the bed, the heat radiating and increasing triggered body shakes—not from the cold but adrenaline. It had taken so much effort just to get to the bedroom.

It seemed crazy that I would be lying there dressed so lightly on such a cold winter's night. Something was definitely not right.

Should I go to the hospital? I didn't want to go again. They never understood.

Ring the doctor? I'd rung so many times before. I don't want to bother her.

This unfamiliar feeling had come without warning, and I didn't have a plan for new symptoms and attacks.

Oh, what should I do? What should I do?

My brain raced, trying to work it out, to reason it out. Logically weighing up all options as my heart rate and body temperature continued to rise.

I took my blood pressure.

Oh, my goodness, that's high! I tried not to freak out.

I laid down on my back. Knees raised, head on my pillow, and went down a familiar pattern of worry—as I had done many, many times before when without warning, physical symptoms came upon me.

But then a distinct difference rose up from within—fresh resolve to do this time, differently.

A gentle whisper of an idea came through, despite the headache and fever raging. It was crystal clear.

The idea, to call out and tell the atmosphere and anyone in it that I trusted God with this whole situation. Truthfully, I didn't even know what this meant.

But I felt to trust.

I might be about to die, and my body might be shutting down, but I'm not going to let it scare me anymore.

I was not alone and followed the Whisperer's advice.

Bursting out, "I trust You, God!"

Nothing changed. No physical difference, and my body had begun to shake even more greatly from the high temperature.

I continued loudly, "I trust You with my pulse, God!

I trust You with my blood pressure, God!

I trust You with my body, God!

I trust You with my heart, God!

I trust You with my organs, God!"

Lying there, I felt a tangible gentle breeze blow over my torso, starting in the center and moving outwards to the edges of my body—as if someone was hovering over my belly and blowing down. This area became peaceful, cool, and calm. This part of my body was not

TRUST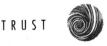

racing as it once had—*what a strange sensation.* Being a cold night, I explained it away. Someone must've opened the door to outside, and the breeze had rushed in. But it hadn't.

My limbs and head still raced, but my torso was cooled and calm.

What is happening? This is so weird.

I felt growing confidence within as the realization came. I had the living God with me, and He was on my side. He had me entirely, and I could trust Him.

I am tired of being a victim of sickness.

I am tired of being at the whim of symptoms.

This thing is not going to beat me.

"I trust You with my vessels, God!

I trust You with my veins, God!

I trust You with my bones, God!"

Again, a gentle cool breeze came—as if a window was open but more deliberate.

First, my left leg, then the right.

What had just happened? Was I accidentally blowing these areas myself?

I felt a little ridiculous doing it, but I tested it. Blowing on my body, gently at first, then with all my might. It wasn't the same. This breeze was inexplicable.

"Lord, is that You?

Holy Spirit, did You do that for *me*?

Holy Spirit, is that You?"

Peace.

The stabbing pains disappeared. So much of my body was now unaffected. Random spots of heat and racing remained.

"I trust You with my blood systems, God!

I trust You with my neurological system!

I trust You, God, with my circulatory system!"

HOW COULD ALL THE SYMPTOMS HAVE VANISHED SO QUICKLY?

Whatever came to my mind to trust God with, I declared aloud.

As I trusted and spoke out my trust of God, the "fan" came over all other parts of my body—until my entire being was cooled and serene. Only a handful of minutes had passed since I'd left the table. So much had happened in such a short time.

How could all the symptoms have vanished so quickly?

It was miraculous.

I sat up, feeling bold and healthy. My temperature had normalized. My heart wasn't racing.

Retesting my blood pressure and pulse showed both to be completely normal. "Praise God! You healed me! I can depend on and trust You fully. Thank You, thank You, thank You!"

I raced back to the kitchen, feeling fully well and hungry.

The family was surprised to see me back eating with them, and afterward, I shared privately with Craig what God had done.

As the night ended, my logical mind began to question and explain it away.

TRUST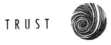

Whoever dwells in the shelter of the Most High will rest
in the shadow of the Almighty.
I will say of the Lord, "He is my refuge and
my fortress, my God in whom I trust."

PSALM 91:1-2 NIV

Did I imagine the whole thing, Lord? Did that actually happen? Maybe it was all fear response. Perhaps the food I had eaten had finally been absorbed?

As I tucked our daughter Hannah into bed that night. I saw that her cheeks were bright-red; her skin felt hot with a temperature. She was feeling sick.

In detail, she began describing the exact symptoms I had experienced right before dinner. She had heard nothing of what I encountered earlier, so I knew it was genuine.

"Start declaring that you trust God with whatever part of your body comes to mind, Hanny."

Astonished, I watched as she experienced the same fan blow on the racing, heated parts of her body, cooling them.

I watched in awe as Holy Spirit brought a similar miracle to Hannah! Any doubts I had about God's intervention as I chose to trust Him were put to rest.

Same experience.

Same blessing.

Same healing Father.

God had confirmed the power of trusting Him by repeating the miraculous healing. We couldn't stop thanking God for all that He had done.

Fear's back was broken that night as God cemented in our family history an encounter with His healing power through trust.

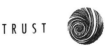

TRUST

— Father's Heart —

"I know much of what you have experienced in this world has made it difficult to trust at times.

I want you to know I was there with you the entire time.

I was holding your hand, weeping with you, protecting and tending to you, all the while knowing if you chose to allow Me, I would carry it for you.

I would not only carry the burden but deal with it on your behalf, tossing it to the farthest part of the universe, never to plague you again.

Trusting Me is closely connected to having hope.

If you feel a sense of hopelessness, trust is often absent.

It seems like a big step to choose to trust Me at times.

But as you do, your heart is filled with My hope, which by the power of My Spirit overflows in you.

Remember the times I have shown this to you, and your trust in Me will return to you more quickly.

You are so used to doing things all alone, and your journey has been heavy and painful at times.

When you trust Me, you recognize the truth: I am all-knowing, all-powerful, and all-loving.

Recognizing My truth is a first step to seeing and experiencing My hope right here in this hard place.

When you accept My truth, the result is always good for you and your future as you move forward with Me.

I don't wish for you to walk alone anymore.

Walk with Me, tell me of your hopes and dreams, your hurts and disappointments.

No area is too big or difficult for Me. I am not intimidated or worried about your current circumstance.

I see the end of your story. I see the next chapter. Knowing this, I have much encouragement for you if you'll choose to come to Me, listen, and share all that is in your heart.

I am your great counselor, better than the best life coach, your creator, and your friend. I am worthy of your trust today, My child.

Talk to Me about your day. Ask Me questions.

As you do this, you get to know more of Me and what I am like.

This will only increase your ability to truly trust Me with anything that comes your way.

There are good times ahead as we walk together in vulnerability and trust."

TRUST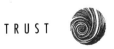

Trust in the Lᴏʀᴅ with all your heart, and do not
lean on your own understanding, in all your ways,
acknowledge Him, and He will make your paths straight.

PROVERBS 3:5-6 NASB

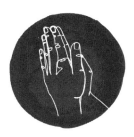

— *Prayer* —

Heavenly Father, to know You is to trust You.

*Thank You for holding me close, whether
or not I choose to trust You.*

*Help me, Holy Spirit, to know how to
respond when hard times come.*

*Please show me the next step and strengthen my resolve
to trust You, regardless of how I feel or what I see.*

Help me to have Your vision of my circumstance.

If I could see as You see, nothing would worry me.

*I would know the way forward and step out in faith,
trust, and confidence in who You are, from within it.*

*Today I choose to trust You because You are
trustworthy, and I am thankful for this truth.*

Amen.

XXXXX

TRUST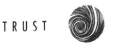

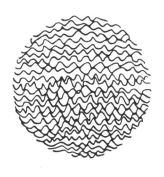

Chapter 8

KINDNESS

Indeed, no one ever hated his own body, but he nourishes
and cherishes it, just as Christ does the church.

EPHESIANS 5:29 BSB

We arrived at the school to find hundreds of kids scurrying about like ants gathering stores for the winter. Jumping castles, bungee run, basketball activities…all were aimed at keeping the kids active and busy.

The delicious aroma of sausages and onion cooking on the barbeque tickled my nose.

Hannah and Ryan saw some of their friends in the bouncy house, and we headed over so that they could join them in the jumping.

It was the first social event I'd been to in a while, and the nervousness had built up within me. About 18 months had passed since the first collapse, and just being here was an accomplishment. Craig was away on a trip, and Mum had kindly offered to be our taxi for the afternoon.

Basketball presentation day was not a low-key event, so we arrived a little later than most. I was hoping to reserve the energy needed for what was traditionally a long afternoon.

This day was important to Hannah. I didn't want her to miss getting a trophy or celebrating the end of the season with her team. I wanted to be there for her. It seemed rare that I could be there for anyone these days, but today, she was my top priority.

I stood watching them both play happily with their friends.

I was glad to be outside where the noise could be whipped away with the breeze. The wind was hot and more refreshing than the trophy presentation hall would be. Simply being upright in the heat for longer than thirty minutes would traditionally be enough strain on my body, so this breeze was a welcome gift.

I secretly hoped that I didn't see anyone I knew. Any conversation would steal energy, and I knew that would be needed for later.

I dearly loved people, but in this season, they exhausted me.

Observing all the parent helpers buzzing about the tarmac area brought back memories of my own scurrying and rushing about during events. I couldn't help but notice the tangible stress on the faces of those dashing about.

It was summer here in Australia—Christmas school holidays.

We'd had a string of hot days, creating a heatwave, which left everyone sweltering and physically spent. Exhausted going into this day, you could see it all over their faces. Sweating profusely, red-faced and flustered, they were pushing through to do the "right" thing.

I recognized it well.

Shuddering. I thought of the energy it would require of me now to return to those times. *Thank You, God.*

Standing at the jumping castle, watching our kids climb over one another to slide down the inflatable fun factory. A dad of one of Hannah's classmates approached, stood beside me, smiled, and said a friendly hello. We chatted lightly for a short time.

"What has this week got in store for you guys?" I asked, knowing that listening was less taxing than putting thoughts and words together.

I stood listening as he shared the plethora of commitments in their week. He and his wife each worked two full-time jobs. He coached two teams, which meant two afterschool practice sessions and two different games on Saturday for two of their three children. They had just finished building their own home and had bought a business that was proving to be a real learning curve. He explained that life was chaotic for them daily. This busyness was familiar to the old me.

HE RESPONDED WITHOUT SKIPPING A BEAT, "YOU JUST DO IT, DON'T YOU? YOU DON'T STOP TO ASK WHY; YOU JUST KEEP GOING."

As he spoke, I found myself speechless, physically overwhelmed by the very thought of all they were doing as a family.

I felt prompted to ask one question: "Why?" The word escaped my lips before I could question whether it might offend or upset him. *Why?* A simple but essential question, and often a neglected one.

He responded without skipping a beat, "You just do it, don't you? You don't stop to ask why; you just keep going."

Something inside me winced as he articulated such a profound response.

I didn't have the energy to challenge or question him further. But I found my heart grieved on their behalf.

I encouraged him to think about creating some space for rest.

He laughed and replied, "When?"

KINDNESS

Do you not know that you are God's temple
and that God's Spirit dwells in you? If anyone
destroys God's temple, God will destroy him. For
God's temple is holy, and you are that temple.

1 CORINTHIANS 3:16-17 ESV

I wasn't joking, though.

This day's conversation troubled me; it remained with me for months after the basketball event. I woke up with the conversation swimming around in my mind one morning. I found it tossing and turning but finding no peaceful place to land.

I began journaling with God. Pouring out all that was on my heart and mind. During our conversation, He made it clear that I too had been like that man. I had created a world that allowed no time for questioning the why of all I was involved in.

As I looked back, I barely recognized the woman I had once been.

She had been busy looking after everyone else but completely neglecting herself.

My heart felt increasingly saddened. I saw how many loaves I'd given to others and yet felt guilty about giving myself a crumb every so often. Before long, God asked me a fundamental question.

"Are you different now, my daughter?"

"Sure, I guess I am…I hope I am."

"Write it all down. What have you learned?"

And I began to write down all the different elements that had changed in just a few years.

Rest.

Prioritizing God in my time.

Eating well.

Hydrating.

Establishing a healthier sleep routine.

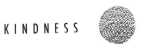

KINDNESS

Chaos had been cut from the calendar.

Spontaneous/fun days were scheduled.

Caring more about what God thinks than others.

Discovering what my priorities were.

Learning about my personal God design and wiring.

Being creative.

Prioritizing quality time with Craig and the kids.

Exercising.

Speaking with a counselor.

Ensuring the Christian community was a part of my week.

Addressing the amount of technology I was using. Measuring how it was governing my time.

Allowing God to sift my friendships, showing me how to invest my energy.

Surrounding myself with life-giving friends.

Slowly, steadily, this list of habits and changes grew before my eyes. These years in the wilderness had been achieving something really healthy for my family and for me. I hadn't realized the power of stopping long enough to ask why I was doing all that I did. Weighing up the benefits of investing energy and time into being kind to myself, which flowed on as beneficial for my loved ones and those God placed along my path.

Looking at this list, I sensed God smiling as I had an "aha" moment. Seeing how far I'd come. Free from guilt at having any time for myself to prioritizing the important things and releasing the rest.

It had been a painful journey to today. I'd fought and kicked and screamed and cried my way through a lot of it. Desiring to go back to how I once was—in a toxic form of living but wanting it anyway.

It was only at this moment, where it finally dawned on me how thankful I was to be here. I was no longer that woman from years ago, full of busyness and activity. I now craved quiet, yearning for quality time with people, and a simplified list of life commitments. Time to process and think with Him. Time to discover how my body, mind, and spirit flourished best.

"Would I have ever realized, Lord? Would I have ever done it of my own accord?" I felt not.

A shiver ran down my back as I pondered all that I would've missed out on if I'd continued as I was. *Oh, Lord!*

"I'm proud of you, My precious daughter. Keep being who you've discovered with Me."

The weight of this morning remained with me in the best possible way.

This illness hadn't crushed me; it had, in fact, helped rebuild me.

In everything, therefore, treat people the
same way you want them to treat you, for
this is the Law and the Prophets.

MATTHEW 7:12 NASB

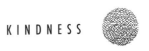

KINDNESS

Jesus said to him, "Love the Lord your God with all
your heart, with all your soul, and with all your mind."
This is the first and greatest commandment. The
second is like it, "love your neighbor as yourself."

MATTHEW 22:38-39 NET

— Father's Heart —

"You expect so much more of yourself than I do, My child.

You run here and there, pushing yourself to the limits of your human capacity.

You think little of Me or My strength that is fully available to you in it all.

You do this because your culture says being independent is a strength that brings you success.

I tell you now that your culture's message is a lie.

Being independent is a sign of weakness.

It takes a strong person to share his or her life with another and, more than that, to be honest in love and vulnerability.

The greatest type of love is to love others as yourself.

I long for My children to stop and take time to soak in Me and then go out into the world with My resources flowing with My Spirit.

Traveling in partnership with Me is the most incredible way to live.

KINDNESS

You choose to run yourself to the point of exhaustion.
Having nothing in reserve makes it hard to help
those I put along your path—let alone yourself.

So be kind to yourself.

Take care of My temple: rest and eat well.

Actively ask Me how your life can be
transformed from old to new.

The new life I provide is one of freedom.

If you are not looking after yourself and
are too busy to listen, how will you have
anything in reserve to invest in others?

Model this self-care to your family.

Let your children experience a healthy model—a healthy,
present Mum. You represent Me well when you love
these little ones in this way. What will they learn from
you? What legacy do you wish to leave them with?

Nurture yourself by coming to Me. Allow Me to
reveal the good physical, mental and spiritual
health available to you at this time.

You do this always by coming to Me and allowing Me
to guide you in these healthy ways. You are not to make
self-care an idol, instead a healthy life practice. It
honors Me as you flow with My plans for your health.

My Son modeled this to you. He went
up the mountain to pray and rest.

He took time to sit and be still, rather than
busying Himself with the never-ending needs
of people and physical tasks around Him.

*He did this with a kingdom outlook
and therefore is a perfect model.*

*I care about you, and therefore you
should care about yourself.*

Ask Me how I see you, and I will reflect it to your heart.

You are worthy of love. You are worth My attention.

*If you allow yourself a healthy amount of love and care,
you will love others from a place of health. Love out of an
abundance of My love, which you will know for yourself.*

*You can't give away what you have not
experienced, My beloved one."*

I will give thanks to you because I have been so
amazingly and miraculously made. Your works are
miraculous, and my soul is fully aware of this.

PSALM 139:14 GWT

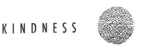

KINDNESS

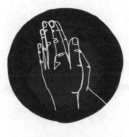

— Prayer —

To the kindest Creator,

*I am wonderfully made. You took the most intricate
of pieces to create my body, breathing life into me.*

Bringing what was lifeless to fullness in You.

*Help me to see how You see me and
place value on what You value.*

Help me to know how to put You above all else.

From that position, show me how to best love myself.

*By looking after what You have given me,
honoring my and others' design, I honor You.*

*Show me any areas in my life that need
tweaking and what the next step is.*

*I am grateful that You have a plan and know
precisely the right place for me to begin or continue,
to be kind to myself—just as You are kind to me.*

*I want to have enough oil in my lamp to be
able to step into spontaneous adventures with
You. This often begins with connecting with You
first, followed by looking after myself well.*

*Thank You that as I encounter Your kindness,
I can love myself and others more meaningfully.*

*Thank You for being the best gift I could ever
want or need. Thank You for modeling care of
self in Your Word and through Your Son Jesus.*

Amen.

✗✗✗✗✗

For everything created by God is good, and nothing
is to be rejected if it is received with gratitude.

1 TIMOTHY 4:4 NASB 1977

 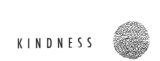

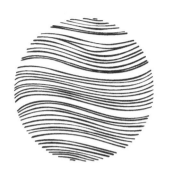

Chapter 9

GOD'S CHARACTER

We love because he first loved us.

1 JOHN 4:19 ESV

Sitting alone in the waiting room of the diagnostic specialist, my feet nervously tapped about.

Would I get some answers here? What if I did? What if I didn't?

How would I respond either way?

Processing the would and could be's, my mind flippity-flapped all over.

The walls were littered with thank you gifts from appreciative patients helped by Dr. Malcolm. Instead of settling me, fear niggled at me.

What if I am one that he can't help?

I stopped myself toying with worries and what-ifs. They were never, ever helpful. A quick prayer went up instead.

Lord, I don't want my heart to be at the whim of other's words anymore. Please protect my

I STOPPED MYSELF TOYING WITH WORRIES AND WHAT-IFS. THEY WERE NEVER, EVER HELPFUL. A QUICK PRAYER WENT UP INSTEAD.

heart. Whatever happens today, come with me. If You're with me, I can handle any comments or diagnosis.

Remember who I Am; remember My heart. Let Me settle your heart with Mine. Look for Me in this place, My beloved.

Over the past six months, I'd been learning a lot about God's heart and nature, discovering how to notice Him outside of the church walls and my own home. He had prompted me to read the Bible with this in mind: *What part of My heart or nature am I revealing in this passage?*

Over time, this study became an experience, an ongoing conversation with God throughout the day and into the night.

> REMEMBER WHO
> I AM; REMEMBER
> MY HEART.
> LET ME SETTLE
> YOUR HEART
> WITH MINE.

He brought to mind one such night-as I asked Holy Spirit to tell me something about Himself that I didn't know yet. It was a fabulous question, which He had given me to ask.

"I am an expert."

I felt His broad smile as He said this with humorous tones. He got a chuckle out of my initial response. I couldn't imagine ever saying that I was an expert at anything.

As I pondered this, images of the best human artists and musicians of all time came to mind.

"I am an expert musician."

The heavenly idea of having the most elite musicians playing all instruments together filled my heart. *What an idea! How good will heaven be!*

He continued. *"I am an expert artist."* And the framed canvases of well-known artworks came to mind, replaced with images of the earth and world around me: the beautiful, the awe-inspiring, the majestic. My breath was taken away for a moment as I pondered His expertise and creativity.

"God, You are brilliant!" The truth of His nature was that He was all these incredible things, and yet, He was also my loving Father—cheering me on in whatever I put my hand and heart to. And He in His wisdom had brought me here today. He had orchestrated this meeting with a human "expert" across three fields of medicine. This realization set my spirit into nervous but excited anticipation mode. God was definitely up to something good!

"Karen…come in," Dr. Malcom gently invited me into his room.

I stepped through the doorway to find a cozy lounge room. Two wingback chairs littered with hand-knitted throw rugs and well-worn cushions. A book-lined wall with memorabilia-filled shelves. Medical and personal sculptures, knickknacks, and models. The lights were dimmed somewhat, creating a comforting ambiance I'd never encountered in a doctor's office before.

His demeanor and voice soothed me. I nestled myself into one of the vintage chairs, feeling like I was visiting a grandparent for the afternoon.

God, You must be here; it feels like You.

My core settled, ready to have some rich conversation with someone who may or may not be able to shine a light on the health side of things.

I clicked back to attention as Dr. Malcolm took his seat behind the large mahogany desk, proceeding to quietly but confidently introduce himself and inquire as to what had brought me here today.

GOD'S CHARACTER

But the fruit produced by the Holy Spirit within
you is divine love in all its varied expressions:
joy that overflows, peace that subdues, patience
that endures, kindness in action, a life full of
virtue, faith that prevails, gentleness of heart, and
strength of spirit. Never set the law above these
qualities, for they are meant to be limitless.

GALATIANS 5:22-23 TPT

There was an unhurried tone to his manner and peace that reflected God's own heart.

As I answered his questions and shared the "journey" highlights, he nodded gently with an air of understanding. My heart was comfortable with this doctor. I felt safe, secure, and (dare I think it) hopeful for an answer.

I felt listened to, cared for, but best of all, heard.

He took my hand, scanning my veins and skin, making marks, and taking time to think. Nodding reassuringly for my benefit, I could see him taking in information and scanning the files of his mind. Within two minutes of sitting down, I could see it on his face that he knew what my body was doing and why. He never said what, but he definitely knew. I could see it.

He wrote down a few notes, and after telling me that everything would be okay, he stood up and in a gentlemanly way ushered me into the attached pathology room. Dr. Malcolm sent me off with some encouraging words and a thick wad of referrals and pathology requests.

As I sat in that room, I began hoping that he had written notes about my case, that he'd let someone know what he knew. I worried that what he knew might never come to light. After all, he was well past his retirement years and the first mainstream medical practitioner with any confident answer.

The nurse reassured me, "Don't you worry. Dr. Malcolm will be just confirming what he already knows."

This assurance didn't put me at ease at all.

I'll just have to trust. Whether I ever know or not, I will be okay.

I decided to submit to the process and leave the rest up to God.

GOD'S CHARACTER

As Craig and I proceeded to attend the list of appointments, we realized just how important this doctor was in our local system. I was given the red-carpet treatment in every test and scan. Being Christmas time meant the waitlists were long but miraculously everything became streamlined and quickened. I got appointments through cancellations; doctors stayed back after hours to perform the Tilt table test, ECGs, MRIs, skin tests, blood tests. I saw ENT specialists and multitudes more, each one confirming what Dr. Malcolm expected. Others were done because I'd expressed concerns to Dr. Malcolm, and he simply wanted to put my mind at ease.

> I'LL JUST HAVE TO TRUST. WHETHER I EVER KNOW OR NOT, I WILL BE OKAY.

I remember him sharing with me, "Whatever concerns you is of concern to me." What a rare and precious mainstream practitioner in this world.

A couple of weeks later, Dr. Malcolm rang me at home to update me on my test results. He could have waited until our next appointment but wanted to reassure me. Each time we spoke, I felt peaceful. God was in all of this and working for my good.

In January, Craig and I headed back to his office to get the final results.

After 18 months of fruitless mainstream medicine intervention, Dr. Malcolm finally gave me a "diagnosis"—neurally mediated hypotension, fibromyalgia, central sensitization were the main confirmations.

Ironically, these diagnosis' confirmed what my incredible alternative therapy general practitioner and naturopath had been treating me for these past 12 months. Now I had a mainstream diagnosis that could go on file. Hooray!

Reflecting back upon this and many other experiences with loving people, I can't help but be thankful for God's nature and how it is expressed in the best parts of us. When I experience someone's gentleness, it makes me think of Jesus. When I encounter generosity, it reveals God's kindness to me.

My heart sang with great delight at having an answer.

Now I finally knew how to pray specifically.

Like Jesus, Dr. Malcolm reassured me that I would get better.

This reassurance and hope were an integral part of not drowning in the walking out of life with these diagnoses. Nothing had changed, but everything had changed. These labels didn't define me; God did!

When I look at your heavens, the work of your fingers, the moon and the stars, which you have set in place, what is man that you are mindful of him, and the son of man that you care for him?

PSALM 8:3-4 ESV

GOD'S CHARACTER

— Father's Heart —

Lord, tell me how Your nature can influence me
in my daily life. What's Your heart like?

"Oh, child, you see the Son, you see Me.

You hear the Son, you hear Me.

You love the Son, you love Me.

*Whatever is true, whatever is honorable, lovely, admirable,
loving, kind, good, or uplifting, think upon these things;
I long to reveal Myself in greater measure to you.*

*Whatever reflects the Son and His heart
reflects Me. (See Philippians 4:8.)*

*To know Me is to love Me. To love Me
is to trust Me more deeply.*

*Just as I know you intimately, I long
for you to know Me deeply.*

*There is much to uncover. You could spend a thousand
lifetimes and still not come close to discovering all that I am.*

*This is the most excellent adventure you can go on in
life to get to know Me and My heart for the world.*

*Experiencing My nature's various aspects is not a
dull task, but a fruitful and fun adventure.*

*These things change your daily life in
impacting and wonderful ways.*

*Spend some time reading My Word and asking Me to
reveal my heart within it, and you will encounter Me.*

*When you know Me, you know the truth, and
the truth will set you free (John 8:32).*

*Getting to know Me will be the richest
decision you'll ever make.*

*As you know Me, you will begin to see the world
as I do. You'll see people as I do. Everything
looks different through My sight.*

*Where before there seemed no way forward or
out…with Me, I shower My hope upon you.*

*I am worthy of the time, worthy of the investment, and
worthy of your heart. This is no small thing to choose
to discover more of Me because there is always more.*

*Some journeys start and stop with you. This
journey is a living, breathing thing that teaches
and inspires, changes, shifts, and uplifts.*

*By learning about and encountering My heart, your
inner world aligns with My heavenly heartbeat.*

*The world never looked so good when seen
through the eyes of My heart."*

GOD'S CHARACTER

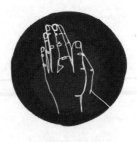

— *Prayer* —

Intricate, complex, and always accessible One,

*Thank You for giving me Jesus and revealing
Your true nature through Him.*

*I love that Your heart is always for me—
never against me. That I can trust You.*

*I'm thankful for Your kindness in meeting
me however I might be feeling.*

*On the ground, in the dirt, or high in the sky,
You are there and ready to connect with me.*

I'm in awe of You and all that You are.

Help me to see You with fresh eyes.

*I long to experience the parts of Your
personality that I am unfamiliar with.*

*Every day brings a fresh, new opportunity
to know You in a different way.*

There's so much to explore of You.

Thank You for being approachable and so close to me.

*Thank You for orchestrating redemptive
elements amid the trouble.*

Show me more of these through Your characteristics.
I know that it always brings me life. You are life.

I love You for who You are, Lord.

Amen.

XXXXX

For I was hungry, and you gave me something to eat,
I was thirsty, and you gave me something to drink,
I was a stranger, and you invited me in. I needed
clothes and you clothed me, I was sick and you looked
after me, I was in prison, and you came to visit me.

MATTHEW 25:35-36 NIV

GOD'S CHARACTER

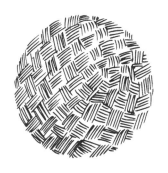

Chapter 10

LISTENING

Call to me, and I will answer you and tell you
great and unsearchable things you do not know.

JEREMIAH 33:3 NIV

It had been one of those rare days when my body had everything needed to live a pain-free and active day. Like I was floating on clouds. Task after task being completed with ease, it felt great to be "me" again.

It felt like years since I'd had a day like this. My heart danced at being able to drive the kids to school and actually walk them to class. Talking with parents along the way. Chatting with the teachers. Encouraging anyone along my path with whatever God gave me. I met the kid's friends. I was engaged and present, enjoying every second of this rare moment in time.

This is wonderful. I feel so free. I am glad to be back!

My mind came alive as I spent an hour grocery shopping without any negative impacts. The lights weren't too bright. The music wasn't changing the equilibrium of my inner ears.

TASK AFTER TASK BEING COMPLETED WITH EASE, IT FELT GREAT TO BE "ME" AGAIN.

This is amazing! Maybe I could go to some other shops?

Don't want to overdo it. Let's head home.

My body, full of beans as it went about all the household tasks others had been doing on my behalf for months.

I cleaned my own home.

I hung out my own washing.

I did my own dishes. Dinner was already cooked.

When was the last time I had been able to do even two of these tasks?

I couldn't remember.

Was I healed? It felt so good to be "doing" again.

Thank You, God.

"Enjoy, My child."

A warm hug filled my body as I thought about everything I had accomplished. Craig is going to be thrilled!

A message chimed in. A family friend was unwell.

I'll make him a meal.

A gentle prod. **"You've done a lot today. Time to rest."**

I am so healthy. So strong today. Nothing can get me down.

I grabbed the keys, told Craig I would be back, and zipped off down the road to buy some ingredients for the meal.

Two minutes down the road, as the tires moved on the road surface, my senses clicked into super-sensitive mode. Every bump and jump could be detected by each nerve ending in my body. Like the princess and the pea, the random rocks connecting with the rubber beneath could be felt as if they were boulders.

But he who enters by the door is the shepherd of the sheep. To him, the gatekeeper opens. The sheep hear his voice, and he calls his own sheep by name and leads them out. When he has brought out all his own, he goes before them, and the sheep follow him, for they know his voice.

JOHN 10:24 ESV

I'm so close; I'll just get there and then rest.

Sitting at the red light, indicator clicking, my eyes began to move as if by muscle memory. My ears became foggy and were buzzing as if high-pitched sounds were going off around me.

This isn't good.

As the lights turned green and I gently accelerated, that same old feeling returned. I was weak all over, and my head dropped to the side. Going at a snail's pace, I pulled the steering wheel hard left, making my way into the empty carpark area.

Oh, Lord…not again…not again…oh, no….

Putting the car into park and switching off the ignition, I sat there, trying to elevate my legs above my heart while sitting in the driver's seat.

The world spun as my head whooshed around like a washing machine.

THIS IS JUST ONE MOMENT IN A GOOD DAY. DON'T LET THIS STEAL YOUR WHOLE DAY.

I hate this…I hate this…. Fear rose.

What if I'm stuck here? What if no one comes? Will Craig think to come and find me? I never told him which shops.

Dread piled upon dread as my mind was filled with terror-filled thoughts. The tears began to flow. Single lines trickled down my cheeks, becoming thicker as time went by.

It had been months since I'd experienced such an episode.

"Don't be afraid, daughter. I am here."

Oh, Lord, I'm so sorry. You warned me. I should've listened. I was just so happy—so excited to feel normal again. I was having such a good day!

"This is just one moment in a good day. Don't let this steal your whole day.

You are safe. You are going to be okay. Take a breath."

The dizziness and tears subsided, but the all-encompassing weakness remained.

I sensed to call my alternative GP doctor. I wanted medical advice and reassurance. Also, to let someone know where I was, just in case I found myself stuck here permanently. If I could only make one call, she was the best to call in a situation like this.

As a beautiful woman of His, she listened intently and reassured me that everything I was experiencing wasn't life-threatening. This too would pass.

Thankful for her calm voice and advice, God invested peace in me through her.

"Have you got something to hydrate?"

"Yes, some lemonade water."

"Good. Now, are you able to elevate your legs?"

"Why is this happening to me?"

"You have low blood volume, darling. By rushing around today, the blood has probably pooled in your legs. We just need to get it back to your head. Can you elevate your legs?"

"I'll try to get to the back seat."

"Give me a call back if you need to."

I wiggled and wobbled and awkwardly struggled to make my way to the back seat. Releasing a massive sigh from deep down in my lungs, I plomped onto the seat, elevating my feet against the passenger window.

LISTENING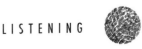

My child, listen to what I say,
and treasure my commands.
Tune your ears to wisdom,
and concentrate on understanding.
Cry out for insight,
and ask for understanding.
Search for them as you would for silver;
seek them like hidden treasures.
Then you will understand what it means to fear the LORD,
and you will gain knowledge of God.

PROVERBS 2:1-5 NLT

What a relief to be able to lay flat and stretch my legs out.

The air was still, quiet, so I closed my eyes for a while.

I could sleep for a bit as my body systems stilled and recovered.

Such peace as I lay there in the still. No rush. No need to be anywhere.

"Be still and enjoy."

That was a strange idea. Enjoy recovering from an episode?

Well, I am safe. I will be okay. I just need to rest.

Better ring Craig.

I briefly gave him the rundown, feeling guilty for requiring more of my man.

He'd come straight away to pick me up. Help was on the way.

I'm so silly. Why did I push through? Why is it that I couldn't read the signs my body was sending me? Why didn't I listen?

The Holy Spirit had warned me. He didn't want this to happen.

I'd chosen it.

Oh, Lord, give me ears that hear Your voice; help me to take notice of what You are saying. I know You can keep me safe.

Strength had returned to some of my muscles, and I felt safe to sit up slowly. Sitting in the back seat was an odd feeling. I hadn't been here since childhood. Aware that the driver's seat was empty, I looked towards the front.

Maybe it's time for God to drive for a while.

Weary of running through life at a pace that obviously my body didn't like, it was time to attune my ears to what He was telling me.

LISTENING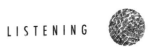

If I had've rested, none of this would've happened. He was trying to protect me. He had tried to alert me to danger. What if I took notice of those prompts more? How different would life be? I tossed thoughts around in my head until they finally settled, and I just stared out the window, not thinking anything. Just being.

Craig's work car pulled up beside me, his face full of concern.

Tears burst forth when I saw him. "I'm so sorry, honey. I thought I'd be okay."

He opened the door and helped me outside. His arm slipped around my back, supporting my wobbly frame. Reassuring me. "Let's just get you home."

After sleeping off the day's events, I spent the next day resting. Blessing my body. Recovering from all that had happened. But also sitting before God, attuning my ears to what He was saying.

At this time it finally dawned on me. As I stopped and listened, God was speaking. I'd just been too busy and in my own plans to hear Him. I determined that I wanted to hear God as much as I could from now on.

— Father's Heart —

"My child, scurrying, hurrying, busy, busy,
busy. All this activity sometimes fills your ear
so much, that you don't notice My voice.

I long to live in effortless communication with you.

Speaking and listening to one another in pure intimacy.
My heart is for you to hear My voice and know Me fully.

I have much to say to you. I have many
mysterious and wonderful truths to share with
you. I have all this and more for you.

I desire to commune with you because I love you.

You can walk through life without Me, but
I desire something greater for you.

I won't ever force you to hear Me.

I wait, ready for the moment when you turn to Me
and talk to Me about the things of your depths.

Even when you don't turn to Me, I have gentle words
of life ready for you if you'd choose to listen.

My words are not ever burdensome or heavy.
My words are comforting, secure, and sure.

LISTENING

*I am your safe place, and My words
are for you because I love you.*

*I have words of life to share with you. Words
that are for yours and others' good.*

My voice sounds like the fruit of the Spirit.

*Are the words you hear loving, joyful, peaceful, patient,
kind, good, gentle, faithful, or full of self-control?*

*These are the things you have to look forward
to, as you choose to meet with Me.*

Tuning your ears to My heartbeat for you and the world.

*I know that you have many voices of
experts and those who wish to help.*

*Listen to Me first and foremost. I will show you the way
through the minefield of advice. I will not lead you astray.*

*My words are trustworthy and insightful
because truth always is.*

*I am Truth. I am also Love. So you have no need
to fear what I have to say to you. You are My
precious child, whom I love. My words will be like
honey to your soul and light to your spirit.*

Come, rest in Me.

*Ask Me to show you what is going on. Ask Me questions
about all that concerns you. Then wait and watch
for My peace to invade. Infiltrating any heaviness
and bringing you something fresh and life-giving.*

*Are you tired? Are you weary? Do you long
to let everything go and just be?*

Let Me be your compass. Your North Star—your guide.

There is none like Me.

I desire for you to have life and life to the full.

Come, let's walk awhile, and I will tell you about hidden things yet unknown to you. Prepare to be amazed!"

Make me to know your ways, O LORD; teach me your paths. Lead me in your truth and teach me, for you are the God of my salvation; for you, I wait all the day long.

PSALM 25:4-5 ESV

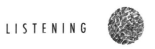

LISTENING

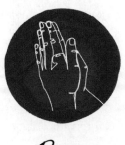

— Prayer —

Loving One who has essential things for me to hear,

*Whatever comes, whatever emotion is being felt, You
speak words of life to me through it all.*

Lord, I want to be attuned to Your loving voice.

*You always speak life to me, coming from a place of
full understanding of how I am created. As I listen
to You often, I learn to recognize Your voice.*

*You draw me to Your side; tell me how much You love
me, speaking words of wisdom and truth in love to me.*

Lord, I want to hear You more and more.

*Help my ears to remain open to Your gentle words of love
and instruction, knowing they are always for my good.*

Attune my ears and the ears of my heart to Your heartbeat Father.

*Remove any hindrance to hearing and following
what Your Holy Spirit leads.*

I am grateful for You and Your willingness to love me in this way.

Amen.

XXXXX

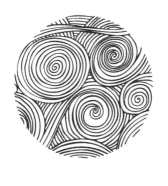

Chapter 11

GOD'S PRESENCE

You will seek me and find me when you
seek me with all your heart.

JEREMIAH 29:13 NIV

Sitting in yet another doctor's waiting room, I sighed heavily. These kinds of places had become my second home.

Like some kind of superhero drawn towards trouble and strife, my sensitive system seemed to be a magnet for viruses and bugs. If someone unwell breathed within a 5km radius, my body seemed to absorb it. Instead of taking a usual couple of days, my system would take around six weeks to recover from each bout.

Sitting here in this room found me with the familiar need for a doctor's appointment for one of the nastier lingering flu bugs. I tried to steer clear of doctors' rooms if I could, but today I needed medication. This virus was hanging around.

The room was overcrowded with people waiting to see a doctor. People coughed, kids cried, receptionists were overworked and stretched beyond their limits. Doctors sped in and out of the rooms, struggling to catch up on the backlog of patients.

I could tangibly feel the air was filled with worry, fear, and fatigue. There was also a sense of annoyance. As people asked the stressed-out reception staff, "How much longer?" Huffing and puffing all the way.

The reception staff weren't the problem. No one wanted to be waiting while sick or injured, especially in a room full of germs.

Lord, get me outta here. I don't want to be here. This is ridiculous.

THEN A MIND-
RENEWING
THOUGHT: WHAT
NEEDS TO CHANGE
HERE, LORD?

Within seconds, I became acutely aware of the absurdity of it all. So absurd that I felt like laughing about it. That the sick would be crammed into a tiny waiting room, full of stress-inducing triggers, long wait times, and expect to feel better.

The frustrated older lady seated beside me was at breaking point; her body language screamed it. She muttered under her breath, telling herself and whoever was in earshot, "This is inexcusable. How long have I been here? My appointment was an hour ago. My husband is waiting. We shouldn't have to wait this long."

She was understandably upset; the atmosphere in the room only served to increase this angst.

Each time a patient was called, and it wasn't her, she started muttering again. She shifted about in her chair, pushing heavily back into the seats, which jolted everyone along the row.

Then a mind-renewing thought: *What needs to change here, Lord?*

I felt His presence more intensely, and a calm came over my heart—the precious peace of His company.

My eyes brightened, and even the "virusy" element I'd come in with seemed to lessen. A weighty download of peace grew and expanded within me as I focused on Him. The result was amazing—like every cell was being injected with it—the complete opposite of what I'd felt in the room just seconds before.

I'd recently learned how to release what God gives to me and decided to give it a go.

Becoming more aware of God's presence, more than anything else around me. I let His peace within, increase, and expand. I then envisioned it growing so large that it spread out of me into the room. Sitting there, I just enjoyed whatever it was that God was doing. It was beautiful.

I looked up and caught the eye of the frustrated lady beside me.

I felt prompted to strike up a conversation with her. If nothing else, to pass the time.

There was nothing mystical about the conversation. We talked about life and social events. As we chatted, others remained in their mobile phone comas or just zoned out, staring at the wall of pamphlets that they'd never read.

I observed the lady, and I found ourselves lifted as we talked the time away. A tangible life and lightness were surrounding us as we connected with one another.

After twenty minutes or so went by, the conversation died down. The lady sat silently, a broad smile on her face.

This was noticeably different from before.

She broke the comfortable silence. "When I was sitting here before, I was furious. I'd been waiting for an hour. As we began to talk, I felt better."

Delighted at hearing that, I responded, "That is totally a God thing!"

She smiled. "I knew there was something peaceful about you. I actually felt it coming from you before we began to talk. Then I felt it myself, while we've been talking."

GOD'S PRESENCE

Behold, I stand at the door and knock. If anyone
hears my voice and opens the door, I will come
in to him and eat with him, and he with me.

REVELATION 3:20 ESV

"Karen...Karen Brough..." the doctor motioned that it was my time to be seen.

The lady smiled at me once again, the lines in her face, less pronounced, looking brighter somehow. She was peaceful.

Thanking her for the conversation and how lovely it was to have met her, my heart was full to overflowing.

What had just happened? How had God done that? Amazing!

I KNEW THERE WAS SOMETHING PEACEFUL ABOUT YOU. I ACTUALLY FELT IT COMING FROM YOU BEFORE WE BEGAN TO TALK."

Not only experiencing God's presence in a room of chaos and upset for myself. But sharing it with a precious woman who needed it. Turning the whole situation on its head.

I headed into the doctor's office, feeling a whole lot better than I did when I first arrived.

Thank You, God, for letting us experience Your presence just then. I'm in awe of You.

I sensed His wide smile upon what had just happened.

GOD'S PRESENCE

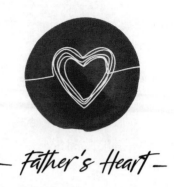

— Father's Heart —

"My presence is My gift to you, child.

*It is a heavenly gift that not only speaks,
encourages, and lifts you but is a powerful
tool for changing what is seen. Aligning it
to My way of seeing things: the truth.*

*As you choose to travel with Me throughout your day, My
presence goes with you—the greater your awareness of
Me, the more you see My hand of influence in your day.*

*Be still before Me, asking Me to awaken and
expand the awareness you have of Me.*

*I will not disappoint you, precious child of Mine.
Being in My presence requires your
trust, but it will be well worth it.*

I long to reveal more of Myself to you.

*My presence is the essence of My nature in a tangible form.
It's just one way that you can feel Me and know I am real.*

*I can be felt, sensed, and depended upon. I am greater
than any double-edged sword for bringing down
anything that doesn't align with Me and My ways.*

My presence can do all this and so much more. I am limitless as to what I can do.

My ways are always for your good.

Do not be afraid of My presence. I will only give you as much as you can take in.

I know and love you so well. I won't ever put you in a place that I have not also resourced you for.

As you walk with Me and become more aware of Me in your day, you will find that My very nature invades all you are involved with.

Things that used to burden you are no longer heavy.

You once had no patience for people; you now find the gold in them—because of Me.

Acknowledge My presence in difficult places.

Choose to believe in Me and My capacity, rather than only what is seen. And I will shift all that looks to oppose My plans in and for you.

My presence is an invitation for intimacy with Me.

It is My way of sharing who I am with you, from a place of strength and vulnerability. I will teach you My ways through your awareness of Me.

I love it when we spend time together and enjoy being with one another.

I enjoy you, My beloved.

Life can sometimes burden you beyond what I desire for you.

GOD'S PRESENCE

*When you walk in the awareness of My
presence, you live lightly, freely, and in joy.*

*Walking with Me is never dull; it is always a
purposeful and fully satisfying adventure.*

Let's have some fun together today."

You make known to me the path of life; in
your presence, there is fullness of joy; at your
right hand are pleasures forevermore.

PSALM 16:11 BSB

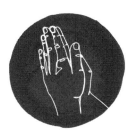

— *Prayer* —

Oh, my personal and powerful Heavenly Father,

*Your presence is a gift to me…thank You for allowing
me to commune with You through it.*

*I love to see how You redeem brokenness and make the
heavy things lighter in the power of Your presence.*

*I choose to meet with You today, Father, and just sit with
You, becoming conscious of You and Your presence.*

*May my body, mind, and heart be aware and welcoming
of Your presence and all You bring through it.*

*You bring a peace that nothing in this world
can compare to or hope to replicate.*

*It is the loveliest of places, where I want to
pull up a chair and stay forever.*

*Your presence changes things. Bringing peace, healing,
refreshment, comfort, hope, and strength…whatever
is needed at any time, I am so grateful for this.*

*Thank You, God, for sharing Yourself with
me through Your tangible presence.*

Amen.

XXXXX

GOD'S PRESENCE

Chapter 12

PRAYER

Then Jesus told his disciples a parable to show them
that they should always pray and not give up.

LUKE 18:1 NIV

*H*ow am I going to get home?

Having made it to church, I stood there wondering.

Amazingly, we had driven the seven minutes to church without incident. It had been a huge week; it always was when Craig was going away. The manic preparation and busyness made it hard to have some slower-paced quality time as a family.

Rush. Rush. Rush. I hate that.

The worship lyrics brought an outburst of tears—a release of sorts as I gave Him my all. Letting go of the stressors and choosing to worship Him despite everything.

Don't cry too much, Karen; it'll dehydrate you, and you won't be able to get home.

It was always a challenge to find the delicate balance between bringing God a sacrifice in worship but leaving enough in the tank to get home.

Life was now filled with measured living, limitations, and processes, consistently needing to maintain the reserves I was going to need for the important things of life. Ensuring a quiet day before a busier one.

Thankfully, the service was nearing its end, so I let go of all hindrances and worshipped without reservation. An outpouring bubbled up from my core. *What is this about?*

Grief.

It had been such an isolating experience from the beginning.

Living as a recluse of sorts. Unable to work as a teacher anymore. Having friends who worked full time. My family members were all engaged in work or school during the week. My time was my own, Monday to Friday, just God and me.

Weeks and months spent tending to my body, resting with God, and endeavoring to be present with my family and home as I had the energy. Being a social introvert, my grief related to my need for companionship—engagement with people outside of my family. I couldn't go out, as this depleted any reserves, as quickly as a kettle using batteries. The bottom line: I missed my people.

So I stood there, tears flowing, asking Holy Spirit to show me what I could do about it.

The prayer team headed to the front, and I felt God highlight Pastor Mal to me. Obediently but gingerly, I made my way up the front. He began to pray over me. I shared a little of what was happening, and a thought came to him.

"Do you know Sue?" he asked.

"Not well, but she seems lovely," I responded.

"I have a feeling that you need to give her a call and have a chat."

As those words left his lips, an investment of God stirred within me. Any feeling of upset left me to be replaced with the seed of future or purpose, confident that God was meeting my greatest need.

We headed straight out to the car. The kids with lunch on their minds. Me, with a spring in my step and hope in my heart.

Prayer had always been something I felt drawn to.

From my teenage years, I always felt a bit weird. As if the way I prayed wasn't usual. I often wondered whether I was doing it right. I'd travel through my time at school or at work, merely talking with God, as I would a friend.

When I entered the adult world, my carefree state of praying dissipated as the busyness and wanting to fit the mold came into play.

Prayer had been a lifesaver during this tumultuous time of ill health. And I found myself asking for prayer from others rather than praying for myself.

I KNEW THE TIME HAD COME. I NEEDED TO STAND ON MY OWN CONNECTION TO GOD RATHER THAN THAT OF OTHERS.

I'd often message my group of angel women who would pray for me during my darkest moments. When I didn't have the energy to speak or think, they prayed on my behalf, and it helped. Often my symptoms would settle down, or I'd feel less tossed about by the illness. I steadily became reliant upon them to carry me instead of relying upon God.

During a journaling session, God gently asked, *"Will you choose to trust Me and talk to Me about your illness the next time something happens?"*

As I pondered this with Him, I realized that the time had come. My symptoms were a little more predictable, and I finally had gotten my heart and head around it all. I knew the time had come. I needed to stand on my own connection to God rather than that of others.

PRAYER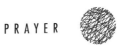

So I say to you, Ask, and it will be given to you; seek, and you will find; knock, and the door will be opened to you. For everyone who asks receives; he who seeks finds; and to him who knocks, the door will be opened. Which of you fathers, if your son asks for a fish, will give him a snake instead? Or if he asks for an egg, will give him a scorpion? If you then, though you are evil, know how to give good gifts to your children, how much more will your Father in heaven give the Holy Spirit to those who ask him!"

LUKE 11:9-13 NIV

During this time I rediscovered my love of talking to God as a friend. I shared the large and small, the significant and the everyday. The more we spoke, the more I relished our time together. He restored my love of speaking to and listening to Him, and I couldn't be more thankful.

It had been months since this decision to travel more closely with God. Getting to know Him was one of the many benefits of this. As my view of God and His loving nature broadened, so did the way we communicate. Prayer was now like a delicious meal that carried over the entire day. One-word prayers or hours spent communing with Him.

I still felt quite alone in my love of prayer. But He'd brought me such reassurance and peace amid the intensity of the mystery of illness. Many a time, He had thrown the lifesaver to me out in the darkest of waters. I grabbed hold and was pulled into His lifeboat where my worries were shared and appeased. Prayer was a gift— the gift of communication with God—that helped build intimacy between us. But my heart had reached a point of wanting human community.

The very next day, I decided to follow the advice of Mal and called Sue. We spoke for a while about various things; the more we talked, the more hopeful I felt. I heard her heart and realized it mirrored so much of my own. She shared authentically, and each word felt refreshing and light.

It didn't take us long before we got on to the topic of prayer. As we chatted away, we discovered a mutual love of prayer.

Both of us were passionate intercessory types. Although that word was unfamiliar to me, there was no doubt about it; Sue was the first person to put language to this. Describing my heart, so naturally drawn to prayer with one phrase.

PRAYER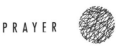

The conversation was energized, and my spirit stirred with anticipation. We agreed to meet the following Friday to pray.

This was to be the beginning of a friendship planted in prayer, basking in God's presence, and being watered by worship. I felt such a naturally sweet space, this new friend, and a new beginning.

Sue and I began praying BIG prayers. Agreeing to skip the small stuff and just allow Holy Spirit to lead us.

Our hearts were drawn to intercede for the world, our country, its leaders, and His church. We lifted up circumstances and situations, but mostly we worshipped God and uplifted Him. Thinking about something other than my health challenges was wonderful!

> WE INTERCEDED UTILIZING THE ENERGY WE HAD AVAILABLE. OFTEN LEAVING WITH MORE INVESTED IN US THAN WE HAD BROUGHT.

We met fortnightly for months. Often she was the lone person aside from my family that I would see all week. I was thankful for the hiddenness of this time. Any traditional social interaction was exhausting. Although the thought of time spent with people was tiring, I always looked forward to praying with Sue. It was rejuvenating.

We always began with brief catchup and then straight into whatever Holy Spirit prompted us with—taking time to listen, allowing Him to guide our morning. Prayer was the lifeblood of my week.

We experienced more encounters with God through this dedicated time than I could hope to cover. From physical wind to answers, to being struck dumb in awe of Him, to seeing tangible breakthroughs, prayer in community with Sue was proving a wild time with God.

I often entered this time, having nothing physically to give. In prayer with my friend, God's presence frequently met and boosted us both.

We interceded utilizing the energy we had available. Often leaving with more invested in us than we had brought.

This prayer time was the first activity I was able to commit to following the collapse. This precious season of my natural prayer rhythm being reinstated was proving healing and fruitful. God bless you, sweet Sue.

Months after we began praying together, my confidence and strength had increased. Over time, our home became a place where random people would drop in, and we'd end up praying together about whatever was happening. It became a place of healing and tending to those who were hurting.

LISTENING IS ENOUGH SOME DAYS, MY CHILD.

How ironic that God would use this time of hiddenness to bring that which counts most to Him and me. Community, relationships, safety, and bringing all that was on our hearts to Him.

One such day, a family member dropped in at 2.30 p.m.; we talked about a family issue that heavily impacted everyone. I heard and felt his grieved heart. Traditionally not used to expressing emotions, in this safe place in our lounge, he shared. His internal heaviness was evident as he looked for answers and ways to help.

I felt inadequate and powerless. *I have nothing to say or bring that will help here, Lord.*

Listening is enough some days, My child.

So I sat there and did just that.

Seeing the time slip by, I was aware of collecting the children at 3.15 p.m. from school.

He teared up as the sharing continued. I felt his pain and felt similarly about all that was happening. I became increasingly aware that

PRAYER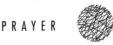

the atmosphere in the room was holy and precious. I dared not interrupt what God was doing.

The only way forward was to pray, so I suggested we do that. I looked at the clock, knowing all the while that time was ticking by, and I had to pick up the kids from school in five minutes.

Midway through our prayer time, I sent a silent prayer up to God.

"Please take care of our kids, Lord. I can't leave yet. Can You just work it out?"

We prayed about various layers of the problem and gave it all to God. We laughed. We cried. We did a little prayer ministry with Jesus. We forgave and blessed all involved. All the while, a portion of my heart was aware that my kids might be waiting for me.

After we both felt God's peace about the situation, I looked again at the clock. 3.00 p.m.! We'd had coffee, talked about daily things, chatted sincerely about the circumstance, and then spent a long time praying about it. How had God done it?! Fit 3 hours of catchup into 30 minutes. I arrived at school just as the bell rang for the kids to come out of class.

God, You are miraculous!

My mind was blown as to how God can move and shape time. How through prayer, so much can be lifted and changed!

Since we have this confidence, we can also have great boldness before him, for if we present any request agreeable to his will, he will hear us. And if we know that he hears us in whatever we ask, we also know that we have obtained the requests we ask of him.

1 JOHN 5:14 TPT

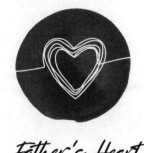

— Father's Heart —

"Come to Me; talk to Me. This is prayer.

*Don't be fooled into thinking of prayer as a ritual
or just another item on your spiritual to-do list.*

Prayer is simply time spent with Me:

Talking with Me,

Listening to Me,

Dreaming with Me,

Asking questions of Me,

Receiving from Me, and

Interceding on behalf of another.

*It's where we meet in relationship.
It's our time together to
work things out and commune.*

*It's where you come in heavy laden, and
you leave lighter and refreshed.*

Prayer is the life source of relationship with Me.

Many have misrepresented prayer.
The Enemy would have you believe it is tiring,
boring, and a pointless ritual of religion.

I say prayer is the ultimate act of faith. Praying
in faith is restorative, healing, comforting, and
connecting. It's an opportunity to unite with Me in
My heartbeat for you and the world around you.

My Word is powerful.

My Word is truth.

My Word is counter-cultural.

My Word is absolute.

My Word and story are an adventure—never boring or dull.

Prayer is your chance to discover who I am
within the word and in the world.

It's the place where your heart and Mine entwine and unite.

Where you come to Me, and I reveal My heart
to you—a space where you and others flourish
because of having chosen to converse with Me.

At times we will talk about circumstances, problems,
and people. I will bring My solutions to and
through you, changing the world as a result.

I reveal Myself and My will to you through prayer.

Then you can declare and release My heart for that
situation, having engaged with Me in relationship.

Through our times together, you will have the gift
of being tended to by Me during difficult times.

PRAYER

*You will discover the deep, abiding satisfaction
that can only come through experiencing divine
relationship as you grow in intimacy with Me.*

*You will encounter the delight of seeing
things come to pass, just as I do.*

*You will know the power behind prayer and that I
answer every single one through this time of abiding.*

Come to Me, child, put your heart before Me.

Now listen, as I reveal to you My heart for it all—for you.

*Then you can pray with power and release, watching
and experiencing all that I have to offer you.*

*You who choose to trust in Me to do immeasurably more
than what you hear, feel, touch, taste, or see. Let me open
up and unshackle the very things which have held you back
from the power of connecting with Me through prayer.*

*I am broader, deeper, stronger, and higher
than anything you might imagine.*

Come, let's talk a while."

Therefore, I tell you, whatever you ask for in prayer,
believe that you have received it, and it will be yours.

MARK 11:24 NIV

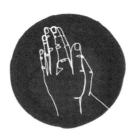

— Prayer —

*Precious God, the One who knows
me, loves me, and is for me,*

*Thank You that I get to spend time with
You, bringing anything to you that is on my
heart. Nothing is too small to bring to You.*

*Thank You for never rushing me—
for never being in a hurry.*

*Thank You that I am heard and valued by
You, and I can pour my heart out to You.*

*You respond and share with me, telling me things
that speak to the heart of the matter. You share
Yourself with me through prayer. I love this, Lord.*

Thank You for being my constant safe place.

*Thank You for understanding my physical
condition and showing me how life can
flourish even amidst hardship seasons.*

Thank You for making prayer come alive in this season.

Help me to love and pray according to Your heartbeat.

Never let the fire of prayer die out in my heart, Father.

PRAYER

*Thank You that You bring fruit from
the prayers of our hearts together.*

*Thank You that I can come just as I am,
and You are delighted to meet me.*

Amen.

XXXXX

And pray in the Spirit on all occasions with all kinds of
prayers and requests. With this in mind, be alert and
always keep on praying for all the saints. Pray also for
me, that whenever I open my mouth, words may be given
me so that I will fearlessly make known the mystery
of the gospel, for which I am an ambassador in chains.
Pray that I may declare it as fearlessly as I should.

EPHESIANS 6:18-20 NIV

Chapter 13

WEAKNESS

To this end, I labor, struggling with all His
energy, which so powerfully works in me.

COLOSSIANS 1:29 NIV

Life in our Cedar Street home had been eventful, to say the least.

The kids and I sat out on our exposed back deck area. It had been another massive week, preparing yet another home to sell. The old memories flooded back. Memories of futile months of Saturday open house inspections. Months of extreme energy output, high tensions, and the stress that endeavored to devour me. It was a horrible experience, and now those same memories built an inner dread of the same thing happening with this sale.

The dark clouds loomed above us, threatening to downpour. Thunderous, black rainclouds opened up above. The flooring guy would be here soon to sand and repolish the floors before the advertising photos were taken. Everything had been removed in preparation for his arrival.

A week ago, the packing boxes had arrived and been enjoyed, as the kids made castles and forts. I looked at these constructions wanting to appreciate them, but instead wondering who was going to clean them up.

This was representative of my waning energy, mood, and capacity. The headaches had returned over the past few weeks, and I was feeling exhausted—a shell.

Where am I, Lord? I feel fragile, weak.

"I am Your strength."

I wished I could accept that, but in truth, I wanted my own strength reinstated. I was desperate to stop the spiraling into the collapse cycle again. All the warning signs were there. I determined that this time, I was going to listen. I was never going back. This time was going to be different, but my body was telling me otherwise. In truth I wanted my own strength reinstated.

I looked at the kids sitting on the deck floor, wishing I could give them some chairs, some cutlery, some routine, and structure. If only they had a strong Mum, an energetic Mum, an organized Mum, a complete Mum. But my body had broken parts that were struggling today. They didn't always, but today the physical pain was rife, my head swam with dizziness, and my joints ached. Today, with the additional stress, and the inability to improve the situation, we just had to deal with what came.

Emotionally raw, I could only seem to deal with what was directly in front of me. Tears sporadically poured out and then ceased—only to begin again—as every little ping and pang within sent me into fight or flight mode. Overwhelmed at all that was yet to be done, feelings of being overwhelmed overwhelmed me.

The children began to argue over something. Probably complaining about using forks to eat their cereal out of mugs—the only things I had inadvertently not packed.

"What's the problem now?" I groaned.

Don't you care? Don't you realize I'm not coping? Can't you see there is more to be worried about than using forks to eat cereal out of mugs?!

I burst into tears again.

Their heads dropped, deflated. "Sorry, Mum," my precious cherubs uttered one by one.

Oh, why did I shout at them? It wasn't their fault.

The guilt rose up. Shame. Shame. Shame.

I hung my head, "Sorry, guys. It's not you; I'm a bit stressed."

MY HARDSHIP GAVE HIM PERMISSION TO HAVE TROUBLES TOO.

We all now sat in complete silence. Inside I shriveled up.

Now I have injured my kids. What else can go wrong today?

"Ding-dong," the doorbell chimed.

I looked at the kids, bringing together a tiny smile to try and reassure them. They looked sorrowful, and I felt the full weight of it.

Making my way to the front door, I winced at the thought of what I would encounter. I didn't have the energy for strangers and small talk today.

John introduced himself as the tradesman who had come to do the floor. He stood there with his long dreadlocks hanging down, a big welcoming smile on his face, looking very together.

This only seemed to highlight my weakness and my mess.

The smile faded as he saw my state. "Are you okay?"

WEAKNESS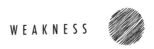

His question seemed to prick my eyes, forcing them to flow once again. I responded as vaguely and lightly as I tried not to burst into tears again. Choosing shallow over my usual deep. Anything more would tip me today.

I was exhausted. Nothing was left of me to feel, think, or care about. I headed out the back again and sat in relative quiet.

ALL I WANTED WAS FOR GOD TO REDEEM THIS TERRIBLE MORNING. THIS HAD BECOME MY INNER DESIRE AND SONG.

The kids were solemn. Having finished their breakfast, they waited to go to school. I spied them looking at one another, no one knowing what to do or say. So we sat in complete silence together.

The heavens opened and began to let loose spasmodic wet bundles upon us. *I wish I could keep them from getting wet, but there's nowhere else to go.*

If I had been prepared, I would have remembered some raincoats, an umbrella—anything. But my lack as a Mum was highlighted and present.

Self-criticism was rife today, and I didn't have the energy to deflect these lies. Today they felt true.

Wary of my doldrum mood and emotional state, my mind wandered.

How would anyone know that Jesus lived in me when I'm like this? I felt pathetic. Wasn't I the one supposed to be smiling all the time? Wasn't I supposed to be strong and capable so that others would be drawn to Jesus through me? How on earth could God use a girl like me in this state?

In that moment of low energy and a few words, I sent up a silent whisper. "God, I have nothing left; please use this body and heart to represent You well."

John sheepishly headed towards the back deck, needing to ask some questions about the job.

I stood up, following him inside. It was at this point of weakness, of nothingness, that I felt God open up inside of my heart, like increasing peace. I decided to just go with it and let God take over. I physically had nothing to bring, but I was in if He wanted to redeem anything today.

> I DIDN'T HAVE THE ENERGY FOR STRANGERS AND SMALL TALK TODAY.

John asked again whether I was okay and what was going on.

I looked and felt a mess but was beyond caring about those things anymore. All I wanted was for God to redeem this terrible morning. This had become my inner desire and song.

I don't remember much of my response. But after I had shared a little of my journey, John ended up sharing his challenges with me. He and his partner wanted a baby and were having trouble conceiving. He was having some substantial family issues with his dad.

My hardship gave him permission to have troubles too.

An overwhelming burden to pray for his family life filled my heart.

I shared about God answering my friend's prayers for babies being conceived. He was amazed. This seemed to open the door to talk about spiritual matters because he began sharing about one of his clients being a psychic, telling him things he still couldn't believe.

God, You are outstanding.

If I was fully functioning, healthy, and robust today, some of the things John shared might've offended my spiritual sensitivities. Yet

WEAKNESS

He gives strength to the weary, and to him who lacks might, He increases power. Though youths grow weary and tired, and vigorous young men stumble badly, yet those who wait for the LORD will gain new strength. They will mount up with wings like eagles; they will run and not get tired. They will walk and not become weary.

ISAIAH 40:29-31 NASB

all I felt was Jesus' love for this man and compassion for him in all the hardships he was walking.

It was as if I was an onlooker, watching from the sidelines as Jesus met this man—how He found him. It was a beautiful thing, a privilege.

A moment passed, and I heard wisdom and kindness come from my lips.

God just spoke through me.

Such a strange experience to know you have nothing to bring. Then God brings exquisite, loving truth at the perfect time.

HE LISTENED INTENTLY. JESUS CAPTIVATED HIM.

I stood there in my weakness and mess. He gave me words of encouragement for John and his partner.

Father gave me insight as to why John and his father didn't get along.

He showed me the source of their difficulties, and I shared with John what he could do about it. This rough and tough Aussie bloke stood there, amazed!

God, You are majestic. My heart sang from within.

I continued to tell John how much God cared about what he cares about. He kept nodding, drinking it all in.

He listened intently.

Jesus captivated him.

John kept nodding his head, saying, "That's right. That's exactly right." Astonished by what God knew about Him. That a "religious, angry God" could be so personal, so kind. This was a fresh revelation for this precious man.

WEAKNESS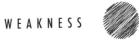

Physically I felt power coursing through my entire body as I stood there as a conduit for God. It was all Him; I knew this because there was nothing of me left at the beginning of the day.

I finished by offering to pray for him and his partner about their baby. He responded excitedly, "Well, that's just improved my night. Better get to it!"

> IT BECAME EVIDENT TO ME THAT THE WHOLE ATMOSPHERE HAD BEEN CHANGED BY GOD IN A MOMENT.

We both had a good laugh about his response. It became evident to me that the whole atmosphere had been changed by God in a moment.

It was a stunning interaction of pure Jesus, and I felt so privileged to see what God can do—even when I am weak.

As I headed to the back deck, the three kids now standing looked sheepishly at me. I grabbed hold of all three and squeezed them tight. They didn't have a clue what was going on but were relieved. Laughing as they couldn't escape my arms of love and celebration.

What a delight, Lord! Thank You! Thank You! Thank You!

Craig dropped off the car moments later, and we all jumped in and headed off to school. I excitedly told them what God had just done! The sadness was gone. The weakness had been replaced by His strength. And amidst it all, my children got to see how powerful God is when we are willing to put our hand in His. How quickly God can turn an awful beginning into a celebratory ending.

God, You loved me in my weakness and mess. You knew what was needed and redeemed so much today. My heart flew as I thought of how God had acted mightily this day using my submitted-to-Him weakness in such a powerful way.

> But God chose the foolish things of the world
> to shame the wise; God chose the weak
> things of the world to shame the strong.
>
> **1 CORINTHIANS 1:27 NIV**

WEAKNESS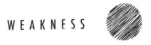

— Father's Heart —

*"My precious child, you were made to work
with Me in life and in relationship.*

*If you are strong in all things, how would
I show My power in your life?*

*If you have no need, how can I display My
love for you through provision?*

*If you are in control of all things, how can I interact with
you and create life-giving plans, bringing delight to us both?*

*If you are good at all things, how will
you experience My goodness?*

*If I allowed you to walk through life without hardships,
how would your humility and awe of Me grow?*

Through these interactions, much happens.

Your faith grows from seed to tender root to large shady oak.

You grow in confidence in My ability to work in your life.

*You become accustomed to knowing when you need
to trust Me for the things you can't do alone.*

*I can show you the expanse of My love for you
when I make the impossible happen.*

*Your weaknesses are the areas I choose to shine.
My power manifests so you and others will see
the supernatural nature of it and glorify Me.*

*All the while, your faith grows and
is further cemented in Me.*

You begin to learn the ebb and flow of My Spirit.

*You experience more of My nature and the
depth of My love for you. In your weaknesses I
reveal the true nature of My heart for humankind:
friendship with Me, weakness and strength,
speaking and listening, hardship and breakthrough,
hopelessness and ultimate redemption.*

*I do not work as the world works. "What is sown in
weakness is raised in power" (1 Corinthians 15:43).*

*Do not be surprised by circumstances that
challenge, stretch, or confront you.*

*In these places, as you look to Me for answers and not
at the circumstance, I reveal more of Myself and ways.*

*I will often use these situations to shape elements
of your being that need honing to prepare you for
what is to come. I don't necessarily send these difficulties,
BUT I love to redeem the very thing
sent to get you off track. I use it to help clear
the path and open up the way forward.*

I am always at work for, in, and through you.

*I am patient with you, My precious child.
If you do not get it the first time, I will
encourage you to try again.*

WEAKNESS

I do not see the failures and disappointments as you do;
I only see fresh opportunities for growth and learning.
The process is just as important as the end result to Me.

Nothing is wasted in Me.

This is the right way for you to look at things too.

Come to Me, child, when you are weak. Rest in
Me, and I will give you what you need for that
moment. Then you will turn to Me and give thanks.

You will become more aware of and turn
to Me when challenges next arise.

You will depend on Me more freely and stand
in awe of who I am and what I am able and
willing to do for those who choose to love Me.

Nothing is impossible for Me and for
those who are My children.

That includes you, My child, My beloved."

Therefore I am well content with weaknesses, with insults,
with distresses, with persecutions, with difficulties, for
Christ's sake, for when I am weak, then I am strong.

2 CORINTHIANS 12:10 NASB

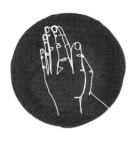

— *Prayer* —

O strong and redemptive God,

Thank You for using weak things to display Your strength.

*I love that You can fill the gaps between what I am and what
is needed for any given purpose and time. You are so creative!*

*You are my best teacher; instruct my heart to simply
be, before You, especially when I am weak.*

*Show me how to depend upon You and
Your capacity more than my own.*

*I only want to walk in Your ways in the
strength You have given me for this day.*

*Help me be content to walk with You, Lord, and
not want for more than you have given me.*

*I want to see my weaknesses as opportunities
to connect with You and Your ability.*

*Thank You that You are not only my strength but
whatever is needed at any given moment.*

Amen.

XXXXX

WEAKNESS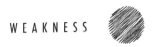

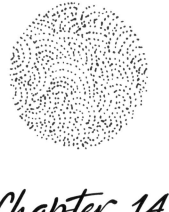

Chapter 14

SMALL THINGS

There is a boy here who has five barley loaves and
two fish, but what are these for so many people?

JOHN 6:9 NASB

As I sat in my usual daybed space, looking out to the street ahead of me, our neighbor's garden caught my attention. It was overgrown with grass amidst the rosebushes and rockery. We hadn't officially met, but I saw her each morning hopping into her car and heading off into her day.

As I looked again at the rockery before me, I felt a gentle whisper of an idea. *"Do some gardening for your neighbor."*

Yes, her rockery could do with some attention. The weeds and plants had entwined and become one. She was obviously too busy to be able to do much about it.

"I can't do anything about it, Lord. I can barely walk without falling over."

Becoming increasingly aware that this was one of the few times I had been unable to follow through with a prompting from God, I put the idea quickly aside; I couldn't do anything to help.

A couple of months passed by. The same prompting came as I sat on the daybed, resting. It came through loud and clear.

"Do some gardening for your neighbor."

It was a more persistent tone this time.

I was still incapacitated. My strength steadily increased, but even ten minutes of gardening would leave me recovering for a couple of days. I decided it was far too costly.

In my heart, I began negotiating with God. I could do the garden if I was back to full strength. If I was healed, then the garden wouldn't be a problem. It could be so beautiful for her.

Complete silence.

I let the idea slide on by again.

IN MY HEART, I BEGAN NEGOTIATING WITH GOD.

Another month passed by, and Christmas was only a few weeks away. I lay on the deck, enjoying the sunshine. Still physically tired, experiencing momentary darts of excruciating pain but thankful that some strength had returned. Thanks to my heaven-sent alternative practitioners, I finally had some strategies that seemed to keep most things at bay. But there was still a great deal of healing to come.

Without warning, the same prompt came, *Time to do the garden.*

I KNEW that today was the day it needed to be done. No more excuses or reasoning it out. Time to act.

My heart beat wildly within my chest as I felt an intense urgency about God's prompting.

Humanly, my thoughts avalanched: *I can't do it, Lord. I am not strong. I don't have the energy. What if I fall? What if I can't get back home after falling? I won't have anything left for my family. The kids are on school holidays; they need me too.*

But spiritually, I couldn't ignore or delay what God had asked of me any longer.

Putting the questions to the side, I enlisted Craig and the kids to help in the mission. After seeing her car pull away that morning, I shuffled across the road to our unknown neighbor. We were all pretty excited to go on a God adventure and do something in secret.

I was so thankful for their energy and enthusiasm.

Help us, Lord, to be able to do what You've asked.

Bit by bit. Pulling weeds, trimming back plants, clearing out the rockery.

I kept glancing around, hoping she wouldn't come home to find us ripping up her front garden.

I hope she won't catch us. I hope I don't collapse; I don't want her to find me lying amongst a pile of weeds and rocks.

A quick vision of me upside down with my legs in the air made me grin. Those brief moments of funny kept me going.

The sun rose high in the sky. The sweat poured. The kids began to complain.

We looked at the overall job. It wasn't perfect; it wasn't even great, but it was better.

The kids had had enough, and so had I. They picked up all our garden implements and rolled the bin back across the road.

This was the first thing I had done for someone else in months, and although entirely exhausted, it felt WONDERFUL.

We all plopped on the back deck with a drink and an icy-pole. Happily exhausted—the type that comes from working physically.

SMALL THINGS

But she said, "As the LORD your God lives, I have no bread. I only have enough flour in the jar to fill a hand, and a little oil in the jar. See, I am gathering a few sticks so I may go in and make it ready for me and my son. Then we will eat it and die." Elijah said to her, "Have no fear. Go and do as you have said. But make me a little loaf of bread from it first, and bring it out to me. Then you may make one for yourself and for your son. For the LORD God of Israel says, 'The jar of flour will not be used up. And the jar of oil will not be empty, until the day the LORD sends rain upon the earth.'" So she went and did what Elijah said. And she and he and those of her house ate for many days. The jar of flour was not used up, and the jar of oil did not become empty. It happened as was spoken by the word of the Lord through Elijah.

1 KINGS 17:12-16 NASB

Oh, Lord! You did it! We got back home safely. We did it! Thank You! Thank You.

I was so appreciative to Him for having done something that the old Karen would have done effortlessly. I felt more myself than I had in months. My muscles ached. My joints screamed with pain, but nothing could steal the joy from what we had accomplished together. My heart was full.

A couple of weeks later, my neighbor Sue was out and about. She wandered over and said our first official hello since we had moved in. The brief conversation moved quickly onto the garden.

"I've noticed you are often sitting out front. Have you seen anyone around my garden?" She quizzed me.

I cringed inside, not wanting to be deceptive, but I was also unsure whether she was upset about it.

Oh, dear! What to do?

Peace came. I felt some courage from God come to me.

As she pressed me further (and observing that she was pleased about it being done), I responded, "God must be looking out for you, Sue. Maybe you should just accept it as a gift from Him rather than search out who might have done it?"

She burst into tears. Sharing with me how she was the primary care giver for her beautiful Mum, who was battling cancer.

I didn't know what to say, so I just gave her a hug.

Sue spent so much time caring for her Mum that she hadn't had any time to tend to her garden. It was a frustration to her each time she returned home, seeing the rockery full of weeds and overgrowth. They stared at her accusingly. It reminded her of how much she wasn't doing at home.

SMALL THINGS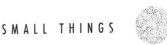

I could relate to how Sue felt on so many levels.

What a brave, kind, and loving daughter she is, Lord. Thank You for loving her in this way.

Sue went on to explain that she had been talking with her Mum about her garden. It was the very day Holy Spirit had given the urgent prompt.

She came home that afternoon to find the garden tidied up. And she couldn't believe her eyes!

Such a small thing, Lord—a beautiful thing to be a part of. Thank You!

My new friend and her Mum took great delight in talking about who might have done it. In this difficult time, it gave them both great joy discussing the mystery of the garden angels.

> IN THIS DIFFICULT TIME, IT GAVE THEM BOTH GREAT JOY DISCUSSING THE MYSTERY OF THE GARDEN ANGELS.

Sadly, it was only two weeks later that Sue's precious Mum died.

A simple act had given these stunning women a little light in a dark season of life. A little joy. A gentle embrace of being seen, loved, and remembered.

I'd gained a beautiful new neighbor and friend through a persistent prompt, mystery gardening, and God's perfectly timed meeting.

What a gift it was in the middle of my own crisis to be a part of His story for another!

God, when You ask something of me, You will resource me for it too. Your blessing to me through this experience far outweighs the gift to Sue.

Since that time, my neighbor and I have done a fair bit of life together—tears and joy, sadness, and fun!

We have moved on from our precious Cedar Street address, but still keep in touch. She is such a delight to my life, and I am so incredibly thankful for God's wisdom and graciousness in bringing our worlds together.

It was revelatory that God brought this adventure to my front doorstep from a place of rest. He didn't ask me to act before He had resourced me for it. And this one small thing brought nourishment to all of those involved.

God, You are so creative, wise, and loving.

Are not two sparrows sold for a penny? Yet not one of them will fall to the ground apart from your Father's care. And even the very hairs on your head are all numbered. So don't be afraid you are worth more than many sparrows.

MATTHEW 10:29-31 NIV

SMALL THINGS

— *Father's Heart* —

*"It is in the small things that I am
continually speaking to you.*

*Time and time again, I pour out My love
over you, through those small things.*

*As you walk through your day and the worries of this world
seem to pile upon you, the small things often get lost.*

*Yes, I can speak and work through the big
miraculous things, but the heartbeat of Myself is
that you might choose to sit with Me a while and
enjoy the very things I have placed before you.*

What do you have?

Look at your hand. What have I given you already?

Celebrate things such as these, My child.

*I have placed along your path multitudes
of joy gifts. They are all around you.*

*Wherever I am, there you will find My heavenly investments
sent to light the spark I've placed within your heart.*

You are hardwired for joy, My darling.

Ask Me to attune your sight, to foster
an awareness of My gifts.

I haven't forgotten you; I see you. I know
you. I long to lavish all these upon you.

I know the inner workings of the tiniest of sparrows.

See how I tend them? They do not lack anything they need.

Do I not care for you so much more than a sparrow?

Enjoy Me. Let's walk a while, and I will speak
to you through things such as these.

In these small things I am revealed in
the most intimate of ways.

I love you enough to share Myself with you—if you
will open the eyes of your heart and keep watch.

You will begin to notice things that are all around you—the
things I have placed to lift you and assure you of My love.

Give thanks for those small things, and you'll
find your heart drawn closer to Mine.

Choosing to foster an awareness of those small things
and gratefulness plants seeds of hope within.

Hope grows and flourishes, producing a significant
impact on your current vision and circumstances.

These small things are actually life-changing.

The seemingly small things of life have enormous ripple
effects. Those small things are hugely significant, beloved.

Becoming aware of the small prepares you for
handling the big when it comes along.

SMALL THINGS

Take heart, I am always at work for your good, encouraging and loving you, interacting in your life for your and others' good.

I do this because I love you and long for you to experience, respond to and embrace My love."

It came about at the seventh time, that he said, "Behold, a cloud as small as a man's hand is coming up from the sea." And he said, "Go up, say to Ahab, 'Prepare your chariot and go down, so the heavy shower does not stop you.'"

1 KINGS 18:44 NASB

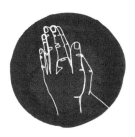

— Prayer —

Generous and intricate God,

Thank You for filling my life with blessings—those small everyday things that, amid the busyness, might go unnoticed.

I want my eyes to see and then recognize the value of small things in my life.

I love that You speak through the big and the small; each one in itself is a gift to me from You.

Help me to hear what You are saying in each moment through the small promptings and leadings for others.

For the small things that I am to do, please help, resource, and strengthen me for them.

In those times where You are showing me Your love through others' kindnesses, help me to cultivate a thankful and humble heart.

I can't wait to see what tomorrow brings as we walk forward in it together.

Each day is a gift, and I am so grateful to You for it.

Amen.

XXXXX

SMALL THINGS

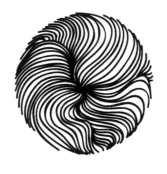

Chapter 15

PRACTICAL SURVIVAL TIPS

Do you not know that your bodies are temples of the
Holy Spirit, who is in you, whom you have received
from God? You are not your own; you were bought
at a price. Therefore honor God with your bodies.

1 CORINTHIANS 6:19-20 NIV

After a string of relatively sleepless nights of tossing and turning, we'd made our way to school. I looked all around me. Busy Mums buzzing about. Those women seemed so "together." They appeared to be able to do it all.

What's wrong with me? Why can't I do all that they do, Lord?

I felt less. I felt weak. I felt broken.

Everyone I saw around me represented strength, health, and independence. It seemed to minimize the small amount I was able to do. Not today, though. Today I was here to be a "good" Mum. I had a large backpack filled with water bottles, snacks, earplugs, medication, and anything else that I know I might need to get through the day.

Ryan had begged me for weeks to come on his school farm excursion. He was in prep, and I'd done so little at school since he had begun. I'd been too stretched, my health too unstable and unpredictable, but it had improved.

The plea of our youngest pulled on my heartstrings. So I signed up, knowing full well that the excursion would be challenging. Being outside, fresh air, slower-paced kind of outing; *It should be all right, I think. I hope.*

The bus pulled up, and the classroom of kids piled in. I gingerly took the handrail and stepped up. Not knowing whether this day would be too much for my system, I willed it to be strong, if nothing else, for today.

Ryan's sweet brown eyes glistened as he excitedly called out, "I've saved you a seat, Mum!" Patting the seat right beside him, I gratefully took it. Chattering away incessantly like all kids do on the way to an excursion. You couldn't wipe the huge grin off his face the whole way there; thus, my heart was light and free.

He was so proud to have his Mum with him. Happy that she was well enough to come. Thrilled that he could have a Mum who helped, like "all the other Mums" did every week.

We eventually arrived and hopped off the bus.

My gut swirled with nervous energy as the bus exited the gates.

You'll be fine, Karen. Take a breath. Nothing terrible is going to happen. Just do the basics and no more. You've got this.

I took a deep breath and headed out into the day. We were a group—my precious boy and his four friends. This was going to be fun.

Goats, pigs, sheep, cows, alpacas, this farm had them all. Feeding an emu was a highlight for all.

The initial adrenalin had subsided. I began to sense a familiar lethargy creeping in.

I hope we can take a seat soon.

One of the teachers made the announcement that it was recess.

For everything, there is a season,
A time for every activity under heaven.
A time to be born and a time to die.
A time to plant and a time to harvest.
A time to kill and a time to heal.
A time to tear down and a time to build up.
A time to cry and a time to laugh.
A time to grieve and a time to dance.
A time to scatter stones and a time to gather stones.
A time to embrace and a time to turn away.
A time to search and a time to quit searching.
A time to keep and a time to throw away.
A time to tear and a time to mend.
A time to be quiet and a time to speak.
A time to love and a time to hate.
A time for war and a time for peace.

ECCLESIASTES 3:1-8 NLT

Just in time. Thank You, Lord.

I filled the tank and rested. This short break was followed by various shows and information sessions. More animals.

My head began fuzzing, and my limbs stiffened and ached. I hadn't realized how much walking there would be today.

Keep going, Karen; you're almost there.

"Lunchtime, everyone," Ryan's teacher sang out.

Thank You, Lord.

The food nourished my weary system, somewhat replenished by the simple cut lunch. Thankful for a moment to elevate my legs. I half-jokingly wondered if they had places to nap on this farm. Unsurprisingly, they didn't.

With the students playing on the playground, I rested. Sitting away from the noise, hoping that the time out might enable me to continue.

As I rested, I began to reflect.

Being here was bittersweet.

Sweet, because I was with my boy, and I loved seeing him happy. It was sooooo enjoyable to feel useful again and do something "normal."

Bitter because this is what I used to do as a job. I missed teaching. I grieved the fun, the students, the ability to invest and help shape young minds. But here I was, barely able to keep up with a group of five students.

How was I ever able to teach thirty of them at once?

So much had changed in this time. Being here reminded me of who I once was. It highlighted my weakness. It put the spotlight on my inability to pick up my old identity. I shook it off for the time being, knowing I'd have to deal with it later.

Train rides, milking goats, cockatoo silliness.

It had been such a long day, and I was beginning to fade. It was as if life was draining from me, and there was little I could do to stop it. It was the most I had done in months. Thankfully, it was about this time that the bus pulled up, and with it, a sense of accomplishment and sheer relief.

Lining up, counting the kids as they hopped back on the bus to go home.

I don't remember getting on the bus. My body slumping heavily into the velour, rainbow-colored coach seat.

Phew....I'd made it....Or had I?

The doors closed. The kids chattered, albeit a little less zealously than before. I noted a young boy leaning against the warm glass window, eyes closed. Being in an aisle seat meant that wasn't an option for me.

My pulse intensified, heart-pounding and racing, desperately trying to move the depleted blood stores around my body. My head swam. My joints ached, and I experienced stabbing pains throughout. These were familiar symptoms of my body communicating *overwhelm*.

The color drained from my face as the day's intensity caught up with me. Looking concerned, Ryan's teacher kindly asked if I was okay.

"It's just been a massive day," my words tumbled out. Thankfully, she understood and let me be.

Closing my eyes, I hoped to somewhat recoup on the trip home.

Please, Lord, just get me home safely. Please refresh my system enough to get back home. I knew instinctively that today would need days of recovery.

It had cost me dearly, but it had been worth it because of Ryan.

PRACTICAL SURVIVAL TIPS

What do people really get for all their hard work? I
have seen the burden God has placed on us all. Yet
God has made everything beautiful for its own time.
He has planted eternity in the human heart, but even
so, people cannot see the whole scope of God's work
from beginning to end. So I concluded there is nothing
better than to be happy and enjoy ourselves as long
as we can. And people should eat and drink and enjoy
the fruits of their labor, for these are gifts from God.

ECCLESIASTES 3:9-12 NLT

An early night, slumping into bed. Being able to lay flat never felt so good.

The following days I sprawled out on the daybed, elevating my legs, hydrating, recovering. Looking out toward the clouds passing by. As the energy was restored, and I felt my blood volume increasing, I journaled with God all that was on my heart.

There had been much that had been stirred up in me throughout the excursion. I grieved my former life of teaching…of having a class of my own…of being strong enough to do anything. I needed God's redemptive view of it. I needed a fresh outlook. Remaining in this place of pining was doing me no good.

Emotionally I was grieved. Physically I was spent. Spiritually I was trying to work out why this event had triggered me. Mentally, I was pouring it all out to God. Relationally, I was happy; having spent quality time with my son was precious.

As I put pen to paper, it became glaringly apparent that I'd not considered my personal wiring and capacity before I'd agreed to the excursion. I'd pushed it to the side. I had tried to live up to others' journeys and had been found wanting.

It was confronting, watching the competent and robust parents run rings around me in what they could do with and for their children. I had thought that this one day wouldn't be such a bad thing.

I deserved one day, didn't I? My body aches, joint pains, and swimming brain disagreed with my decision.

"Did I do the wrong thing by going, Lord?"

"Was it worth it?"

"Yes, because it made Ryan feel loved."

PRACTICAL SURVIVAL TIPS

"It's good for children to know their parents love them. Did you check with your body whether you had enough reserves? Did you talk to Me beforehand?"

"No."

And I also knew why I hadn't. I didn't want to hear God's answer. What if He had told me no? What if He had shone a light on the obvious truth—kids don't need us to "do" or to "go"; they need us to be? If I had asked, I might have had to disappoint my son once again.

> WHAT IF HE HAD SHONE A LIGHT ON THE OBVIOUS TRUTH—KIDS DON'T NEED US TO "DO" OR TO "GO"; THEY NEED US TO BE?

"What is at the heart of why you went?"

"I wanted to say yes to Ryan. He's heard so many no's since I first became unwell. I wanted to do for him what I did for the older two. I felt guilty for not being as involved. I wanted to feel normal again. I wanted to be like the other parents."

"That's right!"

The realization hit like a ton of bricks.

I was trying to do the old me in the new me body, and it just wasn't the same.

What a revelation! What an epiphany!

Later, I was thinking about it and began feeling unsettled. I needed further insight from God about this day. So, I asked Him for a picture of why I was rattled.

Closing my eyes, I sat there and waited for what He brought to mind.

He showed me three aspects of the same picture.

Within seconds I felt Him show me a beautiful theatre. Red carpet. Massive velvet curtains over the timber-floored stage. Towards the front of the stage, the conductor stood, baton poised.

I looked again on the stage and saw a sea of musicians. Every instrument you could imagine. As I looked closer, I saw the faces of familiar friends and acquaintances. Each playing his or her very own instrument.

I saw friends' personalities matched with instruments.

Some were loudly playing drums, cymbals, or banging away on the keys. Others on trombones, guitars, trumpets, and clarinets. There were quieter triangles, piccolos, flutes, and harps. All skilfully played by their musician at the conductor's say-so.

Interestingly there were no music stands or notes for them to follow— only the conductor and their own design. As I focused on a particular instrument and musician, I could hear their unique sound being played. I loved what they sounded like; it was wonderful.

In the next scene, I saw I was trying to play my instrument, but all the different sounds around me made it challenging to hear my own. I was looking about, distracted by others' sounds and instruments. They sounded incredible. I became unable to understand or appreciate my own sound.

My instrument couldn't be heard because I had ceased trying to play it.

The third picture He revealed was an ability to hear what He heard from the conductor's stand. All of the musicians, including me. Oh, what a sound of brilliance, as each musician focused and played their instrument skillfully. The former lone sound did not compare to the heavenly sounds from everyone playing his own part together. Each instrument a vital part of that majestic sound, each one essential for the piece of music to shine.

PRACTICAL SURVIVAL TIPS

I could feel this picture changing my heart.

The penny dropped.

MY INSTRUMENT COULDN'T BE HEARD BECAUSE I HAD CEASED TRYING TO PLAY IT.

"I am supposed to play my own instrument! I am supposed to be dancing to the beat of the drum You have designed for me— not someone else's!"

I experienced a gentle embrace from heaven as this life-giving freedom was released to me.

"I love the sound you make, precious daughter."

I had permission from God to be me. No striving. No straining. No competition. Just be the best me I can be with Him.

Thank You, God, that my sound is worthy to You. Help me to listen to my instrument and be guided by You as to how to play.

— Father's Heart —

*"Be still before Me, My child, and I will
give you rest (Matthew 11:28).*

*Life has required so much of you at times,
and I can feel your exhaustion.*

*When you come to Me seeking refreshment, I
do not expect you to push yourself beyond your
limits. That is not what I designed for you.*

*Come to Me and learn the rhythm of My
heartbeat. Learn My beat for you.*

*It will not look like anyone else's because I consider
all the intricacies of your unique design.*

My plan involves the best for you.

*When My children live independently of Me, their
lives become overwhelming and confusing.*

When you walk with Me, I will whisper the truth for you.

I encourage you along the way.

I can show you the way of life and the way forward to freedom.

*Let Me lead you, so our dance can release your heaviness,
allowing you to float across the floor effortlessly.*

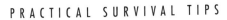

PRACTICAL SURVIVAL TIPS

*As you know Me to a greater measure,
the more you will see My truth.*

*You were not created to always fit in this society
but to be counter-cultural on many levels.*

My Son is a perfect example of this.

He didn't focus on what was expected.

*Instead, in My love, He moved out, resourced
by My power, authority, and Spirit.*

He walked in joy, seeing the true nature of things.

I can give you those same eyes to see.

I can give you those same ears to hear.

*When you stop and rest with Me, I will show you your
best path. You will learn how we can flow together.*

*Yes, there will be hard times, but they will be seen
from My light-filled perspective of freedom.*

*There is a time for everything; seasons come and
go, things move and change. BUT, I am your
constant. Unchanging. Solid as a rock.*

*Plant your feet on this rock, and you won't be shaken. You
will remain steadfast and sure, whatever comes your way.*

*Life will change. Routines, roles, and relationships,
all of these and more, can move.*

*Place your trust afresh in Me, beloved. I
am Your one truly secure place.*

Come, let's walk a while, and I will give you rest."

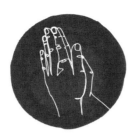

— *Prayer* —

My Rock, my Safe Place, my Teacher and Friend,

*God, You know exactly how to live on
this earth with heaven in mind.*

*I love how You understand seasons and timing
better than I could ever hope to. Please show me
what season I am in and help me to walk in it.*

*I can struggle to understand how to do life well,
but I always feel better when I look to You.*

*You offer Your hand of reassurance,
telling me that I am not alone.*

*You only give me what I need for today; You are
so wise and kind to me in this. Knowing that
looking beyond today is too far for me at times.*

*Thank You for knowing me intimately.
Lovingly, revealing how my unique design
is made to shine in this world.*

*I want Your best for me, Lord—not just
lots of good things filling up the days.*

*Allow me to value and invest in the people You show
me, Lord, and release the rest to You freely in prayer.*

CHAPTER 15

Help me to live according to Your
ebb and flow, Holy Spirit.

I love Your pace of life.

Thank You for giving me a sweet taste
of what life can be like with You.

Amen.

XXXXX

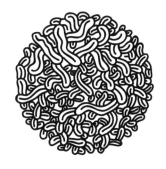

Chapter 16

VILLAGE LIFE

I long to see you so that I may impart to you some
spiritual gift to make you strong — that is, that you and
I may be mutually encouraged by each other's faith.

ROMANS 1:11-12 NIV

I was sitting alone in my car, waiting for Hannah to finish kindergarten for the day. Enjoying the warmth of the sunshine beaming through the glass. I'd arrived early and had a prime location right near the front gate.

Such a precious gift of time—time without any agenda. Thankful that my brain had recovered enough to allow me to drive short distances once again. If nothing else to collect my daughter one kilometer from our home.

As I sat there, my mind wandered, taking in all that I could see.

I noticed a man outside the kinder gate. I had seen him many times before and always said hello, to which his response was a brief nod or grunt. This man was older, heavyset, and weary. His clothes were well worn. Most kinder pickup days, he seemed to be walking around in a daze. His 2½-year-old daughter was a ball of energy, which only seemed to magnify the man's tired state. He waited, leaning against the grey cyclone fencing, waiting for his son to finish.

I watched and observed the mums walk past him, barely acknowledging him, and I understood why.

He wasn't an appealing sort of person. The message on his forehead seemed to say "Go away" or "I am not interested in talking; back off."

I could understand how he might've felt. It would've been hard surrounded by extroverted, squawking women, gabbling away, day after day. Very few dads did the kinder drop-off or pick up. But here this man was; he was the only person who ever brought his son.

This day, I had time to consider the situation.

I wonder what his story is?

I WATCHED AND OBSERVED THE MUMS WALK PAST HIM, BARELY ACKNOWLEDGING HIM, AND I UNDERSTOOD WHY.

Almost instantly, the answer came: *"His wife died."*

Immediately I began to tear up.

All this time had passed, and he was doing it alone.

I was reminded of all the thoughts and judgments I'd felt in my own heart towards him. He had frequently met my welcome friendliness with cool rejection.

I now felt convicted about them.

Within minutes, God found my repentant heart, ready, willing, and able to do whatever He wanted me to.

As God spoke to my heart, it was filled with compassion and love for this man and his family.

Is there anything I can do, Lord?

Take some time and invest.

That afternoon, instead of staying in my car, I stepped outside and approached the man.

Today he looked different somehow, or maybe it was me who had changed, but today he was open to talking. Welcoming someone to chat with, as we waited for kinder to finish.

He began to open up and shared with me some of the burdens he had in his life.

"My wife died."

He went on to explain that his whole world had been turned upside down. Now he was a single dad who used to work in construction. He had never needed to parent much. The wife took care of the kids' side of things. He felt completely out of his depth in everything he was doing.

AS GOD SPOKE TO MY HEART, IT WAS FILLED WITH COMPASSION AND LOVE FOR THIS MAN AND HIS FAMILY.

He was grieving his wife's death but felt he hadn't had time to even do that well.

He didn't have a support network on any level. And in the six months since his wife's passing, the closest he had come to having a minute off was when his sister came around for drinks, and they put on the karaoke machine at home.

His eyes brightened somewhat as he explained these nights. Which were times he got to drink as much as he liked and sing his greatest hits with a safe person.

It saddened me that he hadn't even been able to grieve his wife's death; all the new surrounding him consumed everything. He'd been thrust from the manly world of construction where he knew exactly what to do, where things made sense. Forced into a life of kitchen, kindergarten, and cooking seemed a joyless space for him. *No wonder he was so worn.*

VILLAGE LIFE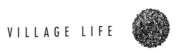

May the God who gives endurance and encouragement
give you a spirit of unity among yourselves as you
follow Christ Jesus; so that with one heart and
mouth, you may glorify the God and Father of our
Lord Jesus Christ. Accept one another then, just as
Christ accepted you, in order to bring praise to God.

ROMANS 15:5-7 NIV 1984

He didn't know how to cook, clean, or connect with his kids. The kinder experience was yet another example where he was out of his comfort zone. All of this was a terrible weight upon his shoulders.

My heart went out to him as I just listened and endeavored to understand. God gave me some good encouragement for him, but I think just being able to share his burdens was helpful for him on that day.

Knowing what the Holy Spirit had told me enabled me to walk forward in encouragement and sensitivity.

And the ideas part of my heart longed to help in some way. I didn't have a lot to offer, but what I could, I would.

The first thing I did was make him a basket of meals. This was given to him anonymously by the kinder teachers to save any embarrassment. At the end of the session, the teachers passed the washing basket full of ready-made meals. I could see him through the glass as his head dropped. He brought his thick fingers to his eyes, wiping away some tears. He was so touched. So was I, as I watched—feeling like it was a drop in the ocean to what this man needed.

The heart burden remained. I suppose if Craig was in the same boat, what would I want others to do for him? What else can be done for them, Lord?

A meal seems relatively temporary.

Connect.

From that moment on, most kinder days, I would check in and ask how he was going. I gestured for him to join the circle, introducing him and his family to the other mums, who, over time, lovingly welcomed him and his children. In a way, we all adopted the family for the season.

What a gift!

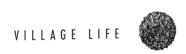

VILLAGE LIFE

Over time, the dad began to smile more regularly. I observed his confidence in communicating with the other mums grow.

A few times, some anonymous meals were left with the kinder staff for him, which moved him greatly. Praise God! To allow him a night off occasionally to relax and catch his breath. Each time the tears would flow out of the eyes of this tough, hardened, greying, sole parent of two young children.

Such a beautiful thing to behold.

By the end of the year, his son had been welcomed by the group. His daughter had settled down (somewhat), and he was getting his head around being a stay-at-home dad. He felt accepted by our group, and incredibly his whole demeanor changed towards us. He regularly smiled and struck up conversations with other parents.

He left that year, knowing that he was able to do the job of parenting, that he wasn't alone, and that most of the battles he faced were common among parents—which gave him a real sense of relief.

I saw him a few years later at the local supermarket, and his family was doing really well. He had learned how to embrace being a loving father to his precious children. Praise God!

We never know who someone is or what their story is, but God does.

— Father's Heart —

"I have wired you for community, My child.

Just as I have my Spirit and My Son, you also have an intrinsic need for others.

Not one of you is complete in your own right, each having areas for others to enrich as you walk through life.

I have designed you for relationship.

You have something within you that is desperately needed by others.

This will not create something burdensome for you but will bring a richness to life that I designed from the beginning.

Understanding that you are needed by others and that you need others is the first step to capturing a glimpse of My perfect plan for humanity.

Just as I created Adam for friendship with Me, so too, I made you for friendship with Me—and in community.

You were made for interdependence—not independence.

If you find yourself lonely, isolated, or without community, ask Me for what your heart desires in this area. I long to give it to you.

VILLAGE LIFE

*After you ask, choose to be open to new friendships
or rekindling relationships with old friends,
discovering new depths within them.*

*Be open to accepting all people that I bring
to your path and to being a friend.*

*Pray for like-minded and like-hearted people to
come your way, and I will bring them. These are
the ones who can be safe places to fall, the ones who
encourage and lift. People who share your heart
about the things I have impassioned you for.*

These are the ones who will allow you to be yourself freely.

*It is not only the ones who are like you that I
design to be your village, but the ones who will
sharpen you, challenge you, spur you on in greater
measure towards Me. Not always easy, but
always rewarding when it's walked with Me.*

*I provide a medley of people for you and your
journey. They may not come in the package you
expect, so remember to ask Me for confirmation.*

I have surrounded you with individuals who long to connect.

*You need to be mindful that, like you, others have
areas that are still being refined. When you live with
love in your heart and grace in mind, your village
will be a fruitful and satisfying place to live.*

*Your village is not meant to replace Me but to enhance
what I am already a part of. Healthy community
will point the way to Me and My life-giving ways.*

Be thankful for the people I have placed around you.

Encourage them frequently when you find yourself pondering how much they have lifted your life and made it better. Call out the gold in them.

Enjoy, bless, follow My leading, and I will bring you the right people at the right time to love and be loved by.

My plan is not for you to rely on one single person for everything.

Each one, being who I have designed them to be, can form a complete community. This will be my beloved church in its perfect wholeness."

Now you are the body of Christ, and each one of you is a part of it.

1 CORINTHIANS 12:27 NIV

VILLAGE LIFE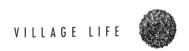

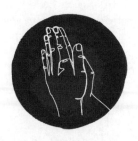

— *Prayer* —

To my most complete friend, Jesus,

Thank you that You desire me to have a supportive, healthy community.

Thank you that there are seasons I walk with just You. And others where I walk with You and the village.

Help me to hold people lightly and You tightly.

There are people in my world who have loved me in this time without "strings attached." This has been a precious reminder of You and Your love.

All community points back to You, God.

Thank You for the people who have cared for me; please bless them for blessing me.

Help me never to forget how much Your heart beats for healthy relationship with one another.

How each of us is an essential part of Your village.

Help me know what season I am in, my role, and honor others' purposes.

Help me to always remember Your great love for Your church and for people.

Thank You for village life, God; it's such a gift.

Amen.

XXXXX

All the believers were one in heart and mind. No one claimed that any of his possessions was his own, but they shared everything they had.

ACTS 4:32 NIV

VILLAGE LIFE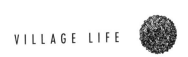

ENCOURAGEMENT FOR THOSE ON A
Spiritual Journey
WHO WANT TO CONNECT WITH GOD FOR THEMSELVES

Firstly, welcome; thank you for picking up my book.

You could have taken a look at countless books; I'm thankful that you landed here. Whatever it was that led you here, I am confident that it's no mistake. This page is just for you if you are on a spiritual journey and want to know more about and encounter God for yourself.

No doubt, God has some encouragement for you—yes, even in your own challenging time. He loves all people, and the good news is that it includes us both. You've read some of my experiences with Him through this book, and no doubt you'll have your own to share as well.

If we met in everyday life, we'd probably be sitting down with a cuppa and having a good conversation about life, faith, and whatever else came up.

We'd possibly share about our tough seasons and our challenges, but also the incredible things—those unexplainable moments which can only come from something outside of ourselves—that have happened along the way. These kinds of encounters are exciting to hear and to talk about with one another.

I'd be celebrating your unique God design and cheering you on in your journey. I love nothing better than doing this with whoever God brings along my path.

I know that you'd leave having been encouraged by Him, and I'd feel blessed for having met you. Although I appreciate your being here and taking a bold step forward in faith and exploration, this obviously isn't our meeting in person, which got me to thinking, *How does this happen through the pages of a book? How do I encourage someone I might never meet or talk with? What advice would I give to those who want to know God for themselves?*

So I began asking God for some advice. What steps do I take that have helped me connect with Him best? He answered me through a dream, and I wrote down the five steps He showed me.

1. Begin.

When I say *begin*, I mean start asking God to speak in a way that you understand.

Start talking to Him about everything. If you have questions, ask them.

Nothing is off-limits when it comes to talking to God.

Talking to God can be implemented through speaking verbally, journaling, or thinking with Him. Our "hows" do not limit Him, He is more interested in connecting rather than how you choose to connect with Him. Rest assured, He wants to be heard as much as you want to hear Him.

2. Foster an awareness of Him.

Keep watch, wait and take note of what He is saying, showing you, and how you sense His communicating with you in the everyday.

Some of the ways He speaks are found in this book series, but there are sooooo many more. Chances are, He has already been talking to you. You might not have recognized that God's voice doesn't necessarily sound like a Morgan Freeman voiceover, mystical, loud, or booming.

His voice can be the voice you hear in the quiet—the gentle prompting. Or when you feel your heart respond to something, this can be His Spirit leading you.

If you've ever felt or experienced love, joy, peace, kindness, patience, goodness, hope, or any other life-giving aspect, this IS God speaking. Without Him, these virtues would not exist.

Has something drawn your eye? Has something out of the ordinary happened? God is often in these too.

Nothing is off-limits when it comes to how God can communicate with you. Take note of those times when you are tended to, encouraged, or lifted. These kinds of help bear the heart of God.

Once you start noticing Him and taking note of His voice, you'll see He is always present and speaking with you.

3. Start reading.

Get yourself a Bible or use a bible app. Plenty of options are available; I have found YouVersion is a great resource.

Start with the book of Mark. It talks about the life of Jesus, and none of this means anything without Jesus.

ENCOURAGEMENT

When exploring online, a plethora of options are available. How do we navigate this with wisdom? I find it's healthy to ask questions about anything I read:

- Is what I'm reading reflecting Jesus' heart and nature?
- Is it supported by the teachings of the Bible?
- Does it draw me closer to God and a healthy relationship with Him?

If it does all these things, then you are off to a good start.

4. Find your kind of people.

We all need one another, so look out for and connect with a healthy local church or Christian community where we can grow together and encourage one another.

Ask God to show you where to start.

Understand that most churches differ in terms of worship styles and some beliefs. It's good to find one which fits how God has designed you to connect with Him.

5. Check out the Alpha website.

This site (alpha.org.au) is a safe place to ask all those nagging questions and to wrestle with the significant issues. It's also an excellent resource for further information about Jesus and becoming a Christian.

God doesn't require you to work or strive to be loved by Him. He doesn't require you to be good enough to have a relationship with Him. He naturally wants to reveal Himself to those who want to get to know Him.

He's incredibly personal and wholly relational, and best of all, whether or not you know Him, He loves you 100 percent. Nothing you could do will ever change this unconditional love of His. It's great news!

I will be praying that your spiritual journey will be the best adventure of your life.

However you choose to take the next step, know that He is closer than you think, cares about you and all that you are going through, and has ways for you to flourish despite circumstances.

I hope you will thoroughly enjoy getting to know Father God in the way He has planned for you. I know it'll bless your life; I know this because I've lived the truth of it for decades. Woah, that makes me feel really old. Lol! But it's true!

God bless you, precious one; I'll be praying for you.

XXXXX

HEALTH JOURNEY THANKFEST

To my supernatural Father, words cannot hope to express my grate-fulness to You. You've not left me for a second. You've revealed so much of Yourself to me in this time; it's made the whole thing worthwhile. The richness that comes in getting to know You per-sonally is beyond what I could have hoped for in my life. You've amazed me. You've inspired me. You've been everything You've promised You'd be and more. Life is worth living when it's lived with You in my heart.

I'm looking forward to diving into the more of You over the com-ing decades and beyond. They say it takes a village to raise a child; well, You've given me my village in this time, and I am forever grate-ful for them.

To my precious hubby Craig. How do I honor someone who has been my best friend for all these years? We promised to remain with one another through sickness and health, but neither of us could have conceived that this might be our path. This past decade you've loved and cared for us all. You've tended to me when I needed help. Whether it be a hydralyte, a hot water bottle, or a hug, your kindness is something that I will always be thankful for. I know it's been hard watching from the side and being unable to fix it, but thank you for sticking by me—thank you for not giving up. Thank you for grow-ing in this with me; I love who we are now. And I can honestly say I'm unsure we would be where we are, without having walked this hard, hard road. Thank you for being the best hubby a girl could pray for and the best dad I could ever want for our kids. I love you, honey, and am looking forward to what God has in store for us over the coming decades and beyond.

To our kids, Cameron, Hannah, and Ryan, I love you. I love you. I love you.

On one level, I want to say, I'm sorry. I'm sorry that your child-hoods have not been what others have walked. I'm sorry you've had a Mum who didn't always have the energy, patience, transportation or capacity other Mums did; I know that it has been difficult for you sometimes…and for those times, I am sorry.

But I don't wish it was different; there are no regrets. This experience has also given us something others don't get much of. Time. Time together. An awareness of God's tangible presence in our home and lives. It's brought us closer together. It's united us in many ways. It's developed characteristics in you which have equipped you for life— albeit a little earlier than I would've naturally planned, but you know how to feed yourselves, do the laundry, and very rarely complain of being bored. You know how to be by yourselves and to be content in that. It's a rare and precious fringe benefit of this season. One which I'm sure will help in your own difficult times of life. I pray that God will turn your hard times for good as well.

Cam, your gentle, quiet, steady heart and head, have been gifts to me in this time. Your hugs are healing; I've always known that, but in this season, I've experienced it. I love your faith, your com-mitment, your compassion, your inherent loyalty, your sense of humor is an absolute cracker. I love that you are following your dreams, and I look forward to continuing to cheer you on, my son, my friend.

Hanny, your joy and boundless tiggerness, your sweet heart in this season have been so appreciated, darlin'. Whether you've made an egg sandwich or brought me a hydralytye, a blanket, or a hug, your nurturing and kind heart is something I am so grateful for. Your sense of fun and natural propensity for joy has brought laughter to my heart, when all I felt like doing was cry. You teach me so much. I could not have wanted a better daughter. I love that you are hon-orable, teachable, fiercely loyal. Like a magnet, you draw others to the heart of God and to life. It's beautiful to watch. God bless you, precious daughter and friend.

Ryan, your creativity, kindness, sensitivity in this season have been so priceless. You've made me precious cards and creations which have brought tears to my eyes. You've cuddled up on the couch and been content to pass the time with me. I love that you ask questions and want to know. I love how God has given you insight into things others struggle to understand. I love that you have ideas—loads of ideas, and no doubt, God will partner with you to see many of these come to fruition. I love that you do hard things—things that make you uncomfortable just because you know that's what's right for you. Well done, precious sonno and friend.

You have all inspired me and brought joy to me by being yourselves. It gives me great pleasure to see you grow and have fun along the way. I love how we engage as a family and individually. I love that Dad and I get to cheer you on for the rest of our lives in whatever you do and wherever God leads you. Keep close to Him, darlings, and you'll never lack hope, faith, or love.

To my precious family, you have carried me when it mattered most. You've prayed. You've brought meals and ferried kids everywhere. You've probably shed tears I will never know anything about. Please understand that these unseen acts have brought much fruit. This book is just one part of what you've enabled me to do with God. Without you, life would be far less. I am thankful for you all, for your lives, for your kindness to me, to us, especially in this time. Thank you for those late-night conversations and the hugs (and everything else that is listed in the friend section too. Lol). I bless you and thank you for all that you've done, but most importantly, I value all that you are as people. I would choose you even if you weren't my family. XXXXX

To those special friends (you know who you are): the prayers, the meals, the car trips, the help, the cleaning, the acts of service and

HEALING JOURNEY THANKFEST

love, the pallets of tissues, the hugs, the messages, cards, sms' of hope, the smiles, the words of encouragement, and thoughts—thank you for these and so much more. Thank you for holding up a mirror to my face when I needed to see how God saw things. Thank you for lifting me up physically, emotionally, spiritually when everything of the old me physically fell apart.

Thank you for sticking by me. Thank you for never giving up—for being real with me and allowing me safe spaces to download. Although you didn't live in my body, you saw enough to know that things were pretty dire at times. You spoke hope and life over me in loving embrace. You showed me what a village experience is like and left me wanting this to be the norm for everyone. Saying you were Jesus with skin on feels cliché, but it's true. I am thankful for you and pray often for God's blessing in your lives. I love and appreciate you, not because of what you do for me, but who you are. XXXXX

To my God-given medical/health village (you know who you are): your depth of heart, knowledge, and kingdom insight has me upright and enjoying life to the fullest possible extent. You have helped this dream of healthy living become more of a reality.

You've tended to my system, spoken hope, followed strings to come to revelations that have given greater freedoms and healing. I cannot tell you how much I love you and am grateful for your sacrifices along the way.

It's no easy path to walk differently from others, but this difference has made a difference for me. You are out-of-the-box thinkers, believers, and doers. Those truths have made this out-of-the-box girl with out-of-the-box body systems a LOT healthier and happier because of your unique hearts and skills.

When mainstream medicals had no idea, you did. You walk closely with God, and I thank Him for you often and bless you in my prayers.

Thank you for going the extra mile for me—thank you for answering frantic calls, for genuinely caring, for everything you've done to help. You've blessed my physical body, my emotional, mental, and spiritual life exponentially.

God bless you with decades more of adventuring with Him, with one another, discovering all that Holy Spirit has available to His children. Sending you all my love. *XXXX*

To my church pastors, leaders, and family, you barely knew me when this all began. You gave me water to drink when my soul was parched. You visited, prayed for, and with me; you tended to me on more occasions than I can count. These books reflect many of the times you invested in me. Thank you. Thank you. Thank you. You gave language to the things I was experiencing with God; you taught me so much about Holy Spirit. I love being a part of Peninsula City Church; it has become an extension of my home because of the precious people who attend. You've given me more than I could hope to repay, but I thank God for you and hope, in some form, you will be blessed as a result of your investment in me in this season. I love you all. *XXXX*

I was given the gift of walking alongside a couple of writer friends, Jane Berry (Ministering with Jesus) and Beth Kennedy (God testimonies). We have cheered one another on, set goals, and kept one another accountable. We've prayed, prophesied, and tossed ideas about with one another.

Precious women of His, you've invested time, energy and heart in this book baby and me. You have been a true gift in my writing adventure. I am eternally, sincerely thankful for your friendship and your fire, especially BIG in this season.

Our times together have been priceless. Prophecy, prayer, and power; you both exemplify these and so much more. I'm confident that I would still be trying to work through so much without your cheer squad hearts and accountability.

Jane, we've known each other for decades and I cannot thank God enough for you and your kingdom design. Although we are wired very differently, I appreciate how we share enough that it makes for a whole lotta fun and sharpening of one another. Jane, you've mentored me through college, you've challenged me in many areas and I thank God for you. Your friendship means a great deal to me and in this writing journey, it's been icing on the cake to walk it with you. I'm thankful for your input, your authenticity and feedback. I'm thankful for the many long phone calls of tossing ideas around, discussing life issues and generally just cheering one another on. You have my back and this book has been blessed as a result of having you in it, and supporting it behind the scenes. Without you instigating the group, I'm not sure you would be reading this in book form, even now. Jane, you are wise, discerning and generous in all areas of your life. You give freely and abundantly, and I sense that God reveals much of His heart through you and your life.

Beth, I feel as though we've known one another for years. Funnily enough God had me reading your blogs, well before I had met you through Jane. Isn't He amazing! The way you walk life hand in hand with Jesus, adventuring with Him is such an inspiration to me. You put your whole heart into everything you do, and I love that about you Bethie.

Jane, Beth, precious friends like you rarely come along. For this and more, I give you big squeezes of thankfulness and gratitude. God bless you and your own projects to come. Know that I'll continue to support, clap and cheer you on because God has even greater things in store for you! *XXXXX*

To the beautiful Mindy and Jenny from Flourish Writers, my, oh, my, how thrilled I am to have been led to you, through Jane. Your ministry/business has been such a God-given gift to me and this project. I would never have made so much headway without your wisdom and insight. Thank God for your hearts and passion, and pray blessing upon you, your families, and upon Flourish Writers. You are truly unique in the seas of writing academies and associations. I've been so blessed by your input and investment in my manuscripts—thank you, darlings.

My USA Flourish girls, Debbie, Susan, Shannon, Anna, Tiffany, Pamela & Annamaria, what a gift you have been. I cannot express my appreciation to God for you all. The accountability, cheerleading, and heart times. You are such a treasure to me. I love your authenticity, your passion, and simply—who you are. Without doing a thing, I see how much God adores you, each one.

Although I hope to meet you all in person one day on this side of heaven, your friendship, love, and acceptance of this Aussie chick from across the other side of the world, well….it humbles me to think of our special zoom times and phone calls together. I love to spend time with you. I thank God for Him bringing such a rich group of God hearts into my life. Who knew that there were others like me out there?!? Lol…and yet meeting you all has been a treasured gift straight from the Father.

God bless you and keep you, make His face continue to shine upon your life, heart, health, and families. God bless your todays and your tomorrows and all the adventures that are yet to come with Him. You are valued. You are special. I thank God for your unique design. *XXXX*

To my precious and God-given graphic designer Abigail: how God brought you across my path is nothing short of miraculous! As I spoke to you about my book, I sensed Holy Spirit saying, "Give her free rein." You intuitively understood my heart and desire for my readers; you created something that makes these words shine. I'm thrilled with you and what you've created with Him! Thank you for taking the time to invest in us.

To my early edition editor Kate, who knew that such a long journey would eventually lead here. I know it was a challenging project, but you bore it with grace and edited up a storm, Darlin'. I appreciate you and honor your endurance and integrity in finishing, albeit a tidal wave of a manuscript. Although what you see here is very, very different from what you edited, I know that He used you as part of my process. I am very thankful for that. God bless you and your precious family and home.

To my brilliant Editor Linda, wow! Linda, you've been such a gift to me and this project. I am so thankful to God for how He brought you miraculously into my life. An initial recommendation for Affordable Christian Editing, a stunning hearted ministry and business. Publishing can be expensive and I wanted to steward it well, considering I needed to do six books, instead of the usual one at a time. God knew. The moment I saw your photo on the website, I felt I knew you. And then to have you be the one who responded with an offer to edit, well, it was no surprise. I LOVED that you didn't change my voice. You edited with such professionalism and warmth.

You engaged with the subject matter and gave me fabulous and encouraging feedback. Only God can have known how the content would speak to you and encourage you. Only He could have known that we were to have eventually met. I honor you darlin, for your investment in this book baby series, in my process and in my life. I love your spunk, passion, diligence and authenticity. God bless you and yours greatly for your goodness and generosity. *XXXXX*

To the precious illustrator Stacey, well, what a process we've been on Stacey. Only God can have worked it all out. The initial recommendation only to realise that the subject matter of the book was something your were all too familiar with. You have been an answer to prayer on so many levels. It was a delight to meet you and get to speak to someone who has walked a similar journey.

Not to mention the incredible way God used the book to bring a little light during a particularly tough season for you and your family. Only God can bring that about. I'm so thankful for your honorable spirit. I applaud the amazing map you've created, with very little input from me. I had no idea what to expect and it's so much better than anything I could ever have imagined. I know it wasn't the easiest thing to plot all the chapter subjects, but you've done it, and done it beautifully.

God bless you precious daughter of His. God bless your Mumma heart and your creativity with a line straight from heaven. *XXXXX*

To my fantastic book cover designer and formatter Steve, you were sooooo patient with the process. Like a dependable ship unwavering in focus and skill. You helped me navigate the waters of an area I knew nothing about. Another US import, you worked with the Aussie girl through late afternoon zooms having the patience of a saint. Again I was led to employ your services, through many God confirmations. I couldn't be happier with what you've produced and I LOVE how you've worked the interior and exterior of the book so professionally. I would highly recommend you to anyone looking for a faith fella, who is reliable, communicative and prompt. Steve, these qualities and more are what set you apart from the rest. Thankyou, thankyou, thankyou!

ABOUT THE AUTHOR

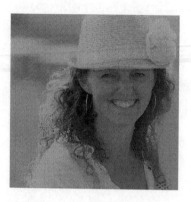

Karen Brough is an Australian wife, mother, writer, and former primary school teacher. She is the author of the *Be Held by Him* series, *Finding God* when life knocks you off your feet.

Ten years ago, when hit by a mystery illness, Karen began sharing the encouragements God gave her via her blog: *writtenbygodsgirl.com.*

Her unique voice makes her readers feel understood, inspired, hopeful and encouraged. She spurs others on to connect with Father God for themselves by sharing the adventures she has with Him in everyday life.

Karen has always had a passion for writing and for encouraging others and cannot remember a time without this. Her blog has been read and enjoyed both domestically and internationally over the past eight years.

She loves nothing better than to spend time with her husband and three children. In warmer months, you'll often find her at the beach body boarding or lying by the pool doing crosswords and creating "healthy" gelato for anyone who might be dropping by. She finds herself telling the family groodle Gracie to "get out of the vegetable patch!"

In cooler weather, she loves baking anything warm, comforting and delicious—often hiding vegetables in sweet muffin recipes, much to her children's disgust. (Secretly they love it though.)

She loves the slower, unhurried pace of life and following this past health challenge season, desires God's peace above all else. She loves to laugh, cry and love with her whole heart and wants to leave this earth a whole lot better than she came into it.

BOOK WEBSITE: BEHELDBYHIM.COM
FACEBOOK: BE HELD BY HIM
INSTAGRAM: BEHELDBYHIM
WRITTEN BY GOD'S GIRL: WRITTENBYGODSGIRL.COM
KAREN BROUGH: KARENBROUGH.COM

We'd love to hear from you!

Has something spoken to your heart?

Is there a particular quote which touched your heart?

Do you have a testimony of His goodness in your own hard time?

If you have any encouragements, fan art or inspirational creations that might help inspire or affirm others, share and connect with your online village on the

'Be Held by Him' facebook page

or email us at beheldbyhimseries@gmail.com

GOD BLESS YOU DEARLY, BRAVE ONE.

Next in the series:

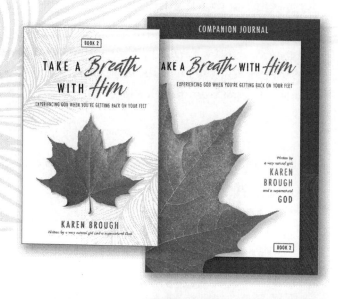

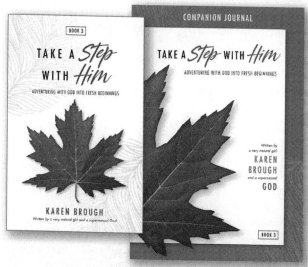

Made in the USA
Columbia, SC
08 November 2024

46011315R00159